An Introduction to Community Medicine

CHURCHILL LIVINGSTONE
MEDICAL TEXTS

Notes on Infectious Diseases
Edited by *A.P. Ball*

Epidemiology in Medical Practice
Second edition
D.J.P. Barker and G. Rose

Pain: Its Nature, Analysis and Treatment
Michael R. Bond

Geriatric Medicine for Students
Second edition
J.C. Brocklehurst and T. Hanley

Essentials of Dermatology
J.L. Burton

Essential Ophthalmology
Hector Bryson Chawla

An Introduction to Clinical Rheumatology
Second edition
William Cabon Dick

Sexual Problems and their Management
C. Fairburn, M. Dickerson and J. Greenwood

Notes on Psychiatry Fifth edition
I.M. Ingram, G.C. Timbury and R.M. Mowbray

Elements of Medical Genetics
Sixth edition
Alan E.H. Emery

Physiology: A Clinical Approach
Third edition
G.R. Kelman

A Concise Textbook of Gastroenterology
Second edition
M.J.S. Langman

Tumours: Basic Principles and Clinical Aspects
Christopher Louis

Nutrition and its Disorders
Third edition
Donald S. McLaren

Introduction to Clinical Examination
Third edition
J. Macleod, E.B. French and J.F. Munro

The Essentials of Neuroanatomy
Fourth edition
G.A.G. Mitchell and D. Mayor

An Introduction to Primary Medical Care
Second edition
D.C. Morrell

Urology and Renal Medicine
Third edition
J.E. Newsam and J.J.B. Petrie

Clinical Bacteriology
P.W. Ross

Sexually Transmitted Diseases
Third edition
C.B.S. Schofield

Notes on Medical Bacteriology
J.D. Sleigh and Morag C. Timbury

An Introduction to General Pathology
Second edition
W.G. Spector

Child Psychiatry for Students
Second edition
Frederick H. Stone and Cyrille Koupernik

Introduction to Clinical Endocrinology
Second edition
John A. Thomson

Notes on Medical Virology
Seventh edition
Morag C. Timbury

Clinical Pharmacology
Fourth edition
P. Turner and A. Richens

Immunology: An Outline for Students of Medicine and Biology
Fifth edition
D.M. Weir

Essentials of Obstetrics and Gynaeology
Second edition
James Willocks

Clinical Thinking and Practice: Diagnosis and Decision in Patient Care
H.J. Wright and D.B. MacAdam

LIVINGSTONE MEDICAL TEXTS

Psychological Medicine for Students
John Pollitt

Respiratory Medicine *Malcolm Schonell*

Cardiology for Students *Max Zoob*

An Introduction to Community Medicine

Charles du V. Florey MD MPH FFCM
Professor of Community Medicine

Peter Burney MA MB BS
Lecturer in Community Medicine

Michael D'Souza MD MRCGP MFCM
Principal in General Practice

Ellie Scrivens BA
Lecturer in Social Administration

Peter West DPhil
Senior Lecturer in Health Economics

Department of Community Medicine,
St Thomas' Hospital Medical School,
London

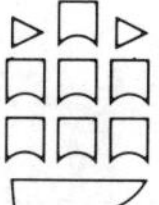

CHURCHILL LIVINGSTONE
EDINBURGH LONDON MELBOURNE AND NEW YORK 1983

CHURCHILL LIVINGSTONE
Medical Division of Longman Group Limited

Distributed in the United States of America by Churchill Livingstone Inc., 1560 Broadway, New York, N.Y. 10036, and by associated companies, branches and representatives throughout the world.

First published 1983

ISBN 0 443 02464 2

British Library Cataloguing in Publication Data
An Introduction to community medicine. —
(Churchill Livingstone medical text)
1. Community health services — Great Britain
I. Title II. Florey, Charles du V.
III. Series
362.1'0425 RA485

Library of Congress Cataloging in Publication Data
An Introduction to community medicine.
(Churchill Livingstone medical text)
Includes index.
1. Community health services. 2. Public health.
I. Florey, Charles du V. II. Title: Community medicine.
III. Series. [DNLM: 1. Community Medicine.
W 84.5 161]
RA425.157 1983 362.1'2 82-22064

Printed in Singapore by Huntsmen Offset Printing Pte Ltd

Preface

Community Medicine came of age in the United Kingdom in 1974 with the reorganisation of the National Health Service. Until that time such terms as 'Public Health' or 'Social Medicine' had been used and their meaning was generally agreed. However, 'Community Medicine' is a term which still confuses, as its scope is neither obvious nor the same from one country to another. Here we use it to cover a specialty concerned with the care of groups rather than individuals, thus excluding the individual care given by general practitioners but including, for example, the immunisation of populations in which general practitioners play a role.

In this introduction to community medicine our intention is to give an overview of the subject in as far as we can within the limited space. We have tried to provide the essentials of the subject by introducing central concepts without undue stress on the more ephemeral aspects of management structure or 'established truth'.

The book is designed to be read from the beginning. The plot involves the life of a problem, its epidemiological unravelling, assessment of the answer and the implementation of a solution through policy making and management systems. It incorporates the bare bones of the mixture of academic and service community medicine: we have intentionally omitted some areas which might be thought fundamental to community medicine such as the structure and function of the NHS. We have tried to emphasise ideas and concepts that lie behind the practice of community medicine rather than 'facts', particularly when the latter are prone to rapid change. We are also aware that we have omitted other areas in which community physicians should have competence, but which are not central to our theme.

The book is primarily directed towards medical students and is thus a general view of the subject. Within it they are introduced to the epidemiological approach, the measurement of effectiveness and efficiency in health care, a framework for thought on medical economics and an appreciation of the difficulties of introducing change into a health system. There are already many books on facets of community medicine both covered and untouched in this volume: we hope that the particular combination chosen here may give a new perspective to the subject.

We would like to thank Professor John Colley and Professor Walter Holland for their many helpful comments on the text. We would also like to thank all the members of our department who gave so willingly of their time to read and advise on each draft and to thank the secretaries who spent more hours at the word processor than we could count.

London 1983

Charles du V. Florey
Peter Burney
Michael D'Souza
Ellie Scrivens
Peter West

Contents

1

Introduction

The practice of medicine traditionally involves a one to one relationship between patient and doctor. The doctor's role is to provide cure, care and compassion in an attempt to reverse or stem the progress of an individual's disease. This is the core of most current medical education, but it tends to exclude the broader view of the community from which the patients come and it limits both the study of disease aetiology and the creation of preventive strategies. Community medicine is the specialty in which medical science is applied to groups and populations rather than to individuals. It requires techniques and a philosophy which, although they frequently differ from those used in clinical practice, can raise the satisfaction to be had from clinical medicine through a deeper understanding of health and illness.

There are three major areas in which study of the health of groups has advantages over the study of individual patients: the estimation of biological variability, the discovery of factors which predispose to disease and which may be altered by preventive action, and the planning of health services.

Biological variability

Biological variability is used here to mean the variation that exists between people in characteristics such as height, heart size, red cell count or intelligence quotient. Although observations made on a single individual may give insight into a problem, they are rarely suitable for drawing firm conclusions about the characteristics either of a particular group of people—patients with some disease—or about the differences between patients and healthy people. A single case study may suggest that the patient's disease is related to some previous experience or exposure, but it cannot show whether the experience is just as common among healthy people. A single patient with lung cancer who smokes heavily does not show that smoking causes lung cancer, but the causal association becomes more certain if lung cancer is found to be rare in non-smoking groups of people and increasingly common in groups smoking increasing amounts of tobacco. Similarly, a single fasting blood glucose measurement cannot be interpreted without reference to the range of values to be expected in a group of non-diabetics, and the diagnosis of hypertension can only be based on what is known about the range, or distribution, of blood pressure in the general population and about the levels which predict future morbid events such as myocardial infarction or cerebral stroke. If a single patient with breast cancer survives for 10 years on Laetrile, the efficacy of the treatment is not proven since survival of patients without treatment varies greatly and may also exceed 10 years.

Information drawn from the study of groups is used by the clinician to make a diagnosis, to assess prognosis and to prescribe treatment. Symptoms, signs and past medical history will play an important part in determining the differential diagnosis, and other personal factors may also be used. A clinician will consider the patient's age, sex, ethnic group, marital status and social class which are all related in different ways to different conditions. He may also find the patient's occupation and smoking, drinking and eating habits useful in reaching a diagnosis.

Although he may not always think of it in arithmetic terms, his choice of diagnosis involves estimating the likelihood that the observations he has made on his patient are due to each of his differential diagnoses. Such probabilities can only be estimated from observations on groups: they may come from his own knowledge of the patients in his practice, they may come from what he has read or heard of current epidemics of infectious diseases or they may come from his understanding of epidemiological studies. He makes best use of these probabilities if he knows how they were obtained and to what extent they may be in error, that is, if he has an understanding of the principles of epidemiology and medical statistics.

The origins of disease and prevention

A major premise of community medicine is that the origins of disease lie in part in the way we live. It is in recognition of this that clinicians take a social and occupational history from their patients. A further premise is that health can be fostered and disease prevented by improving the social and physical environment, but it is only rarely possible to change the circumstances of people's lives by dealing with them as isolated individuals.

One problem with an individual approach is that personal habits are rarely established by individual choice. Man is a great conformist. To take one example, dietary habits are largely prescribed by culture. The slow virus of 'Kuru' was transmitted by the custom among the South Fore people of Papua New Guinea of eating raw human brains on certain ceremonial occasions. Beef tapeworm is transmitted more commonly where raw beef is eaten, as in steak tartare, popular in France. A number of gastrointestinal diseases are more common in the industrialised West where a low residue diet is eaten. All three of these dietary habits are in their way harmful and none has any rational justification to an outsider, but where they are the custom they are difficult for the individual to discard.

During the Second World War, meat and other protein were very scarce in the UK but, despite the extreme conditions of war-time, there was considerable resistance to the idea of eating animals such as horses that were not generally thought of as 'food'. This reluctance to use alternative sources of nutrition remains a problem in many of the poorer countries today. The same reluctance to change is seen in industrialised countries where the introduction of a prudent diet for the prevention of heart disease has been generally unsuccessful because of the major switch in composition required from the usual diet.

Furthermore, individuals are often unable to control their own environment. If a man abstains from alcohol when driving, he reduces his risk of being involved in an accident. But if the custom is to drink and drive, his chances of meeting with an accident because some other driver is inebriated, even if he is sober, are still high. In the same way, an individual can do very little about the quality of the air he breathes out of doors, because this is more influenced by what other people do.

There are thus certain social and environmental factors affecting health that are beyond the control of the individual; if these are to be changed, they must be changed for everyone.

The need to plan health services

When a doctor sets up in practice he may attract a clientele and, according to his reputation, may obtain more work than he can manage. In the normal course of clinical practice he has little need to plan his services in order to do the work for which he was trained and to offer to the majority of individuals who consult him an excellent personal service. From the individual doctor's point of view this may seem adequate, but a wider view may give a different picture. In community medicine some account must also be taken of those who are not treated and who perhaps do not come to the doctor. If a doctor spends a great deal of time with one group of patients, they may agree that he is successful; but if this success excludes other groups from care, there are grounds for questioning whether the best use is being made of his time.

To overcome this problem, health services need to be organised in some way: the distribution of health manpower and finance may be decided by market forces as in the example above or by central planning. The argument against central planning is based to some extent on the liberal assumption of classical economic theory that if free choice is maximised, people choose what is best for them. If a good service is provided at a reasonable cost that service will flourish, as will those who provide it. At the same time those who provide a poor service will have to change their ways or turn to some other business. Thus the power of the market provides the maximum benefit for all. This was described by Adam Smith as the 'invisible hand' of the free market.

But health services are not like other marketable services. The greatest burden of ill health falls on the poor which means that in the free market those who have the most need of services are those who are least able to obtain them. At least in industrial societies good health is seen as a right rather than a luxury and therefore governments feel compelled to intervene. They may either provide some form of income supplement or health insurance scheme for the poor and the elderly, as in the USA, or provide a centrally planned health service at nominal charge, as in the UK.

If there is a centrally planned service there is no 'invisible hand' to plan health services by default, and decisions have to be made on their optimal distribution. These decisions must be based on information about the distribution of diseases, the effectiveness of different methods of dealing with those diseases, and the costs of the different options. Although a political judgement will be required to make a final decision between all the possible choices, this judgement should be properly informed.

The community physician: epidemiologist and planner

Before the reorganisation of the health services in 1974, the local authorities employed Medical Officers of Health to advise on issues of public health. Their traditional areas of interest were infectious disease control and child health but expansion of the National Health Service and the decline of infectious disease made this role obsolete. In the reorganisation of the health services the importance of applying the disciplines of epidemiology and medical statistics to the planning of services as well as to the outbreak of epidemics was recognised in the establishment of the post of District Community Physician (District Medical Officer since the reorganisation in

1982). These officers are appointed as members of the management teams in each District, with an equivalent post held on the management teams at Area and Region (Areas were discontinued in 1982). They are responsible for advising the management team on epidemiological issues and also on planning services. They also have management responsibilities with the National Health Service and an obligation to ensure adequate liason and coordination of services. In addition, there are Specialists in Community Medicine who are removed from the management structure of the Health Service. They have specialist jobs in a number of fields including 'Information and Planning' and 'Child Health'. In a consultant capacity, they provide expert advice to the managers of the health services.

Plan of the book

Community medicine covers many activities and interests. Its basic scientific disciplines are epidemiology and medical statistics and its service role is the application of epidemiology to the prevention of disease and the planning and coordination of health services. In this book we have first tried to show how the epidemiological method can be used to describe problems in the community and to determine the risk factors for disease. This provides the background for a discussion of the options for disease control and the strategies for the evaluation of treatment and health services. The multidisciplinary nature of community medicine becomes evident in the explanation of the economic methods used to determine which services to offer. The final chapter discusses the problems of policy formation, planning and management in a service in which clinicians can still retain the maximum freedom to treat their patients as they see best.

2

The origin of health problems in the community

Throughout human history the origin of health problems has been a subject for recurrent hypothesis and speculation.

Ill health has been traditionally attributed to two main causes, namely invasion of the individual by harmful external agents, and disturbances arising within the individual.

We have come to recognise that, although there are instances in which only one type of cause operates, as in overwhelming poisoning or serious genetic disorder, in general, ill health is due to the interplay between both external and internal factors.

While the intensive study of the pathophysiology of sick individuals often suggests causative factors which might be relevant, only when we study whole families or whole communities and in particular, when we do intervention trials, can we demonstrate which factors are of general aetiological importance. The community approach to the problem of ill health is that of the broad view in which the whole population becomes 'the patient' and concern is with the group rather than the individual. In addition, just as the study of both normal and diseased cells underlies any understanding of the clinical problems of the sick individual, the study of both healthy and sick individuals underlies the understanding of community medicine.

THE DEFINITION OF HEALTH PROBLEMS

When ill health is viewed *solely* from the viewpoint of the individual, it is simply his own experience of certain unpleasant symptoms. This purely subjective type of ill health may be termed 'illness'. When an illness is taken to others for help it may be termed a 'complaint', and when an individual's complaint is of sufficient severity to excuse him from social obligations then it may be termed 'sickness'. However, only when a condition is labelled or diagnosed by a doctor can it be termed 'disease'. In recent times, it has become clear from the screening of whole populations that a large amount of disease goes unrecognised and much illness is never seen by a doctor. The model of the iceberg has been used to describe the totality of health problems and the term 'health problem' is perhaps the most useful to describe all forms of illness, complaint, sickness and disease whether it is in the exposed or submerged part of the iceberg.

THE VALUE OF A COMMUNITY VIEW OF HEALTH

An understanding of how health problems affect groups governs a great deal of current medical practice because the received wisdom which forms the basis of medical teaching is usually derived both from our clinical experience of treating many patients and from formal group experiments such as trials. When we look at the scale and severity of health problems within a community it is possible to study their components separately and to observe where and when they overlap.

Such an overview of community ill health is not only valuable for the planning of health services but also affords a fresh perspective for the administration of sensible and sensitive personal medical care. It may, for instance, prevent doctors attempting to deal with problems that are best left in the ambit of the counsellor or social worker and alert them to the social origins of ill health. Indeed the importance of doctors acquiring a community view of health as opposed to merely studying the sick individual has been steadily increasing. For example, cholera was the first disease to be recognised as having a cause intimately related to the way communities functioned with respect to their water supplies and sanitation. This realisation by John Snow did much to establish the discipline of epidemiology and replaced inadequate treatment of severely diseased individuals with highly effective preventive care for communities. That public health measures such as improving water supplies and sanitation have since saved more lives than the ordinary practice of clinical medicine is now beyond reasonable doubt.

Today, the changing state of the industrial urban environment, in which over 80 per cent of the population of the developed world live, is creating whole new categories of illnesses and diseases. Television epilepsy, tolylene diisocyanate asthma and tartrazine urticaria are just a few examples of illnesses which are a product of the modern environment. Thus a community view of health problems can lead to both the recognition of diseases and their causes and may guide our interventions to achieve better health.

DESCRIPTIVE INFORMATION ABOUT HEALTH PROBLEMS

Most countries routinely collect information on the size of their population and many of its characteristics including its health. This information is by no means exhaustive nor is it invariably accurate. Data on population size are derived from the population census, the registration of births and deaths and immigration and emigration statistics. For some countries such as China and India the task of registration has so far proved too onerous and expensive to be implemented but in most developed countries these procedures have been instituted over many years and provide the basis for useful international comparisons.

Mortality

In the UK the Government publishes a large amount of information about health problems. The Office of Population Censuses and Surveys (OPCS) publishes statistics annually which give overall figures for births and deaths comparing local with national rates. Also published are deaths by cause within sex and age groups. Major sources of inaccuracy in these data are diagnostic errors by doctors who complete the death certificates and administrative errors in determining population size. However mortality data provide probably the most complete routinely available information about the underlying health of the population.

From such data it is possible to get an overall picture of the major groups of conditions that cause death in the UK (Table 2.1), classified using the International Classification of Diseases (ICD).

Cardiovascular disease and neoplasms are the two most commonly certified causes of death. They account for two-thirds of all mortality. They are much more common in old age and indeed 72 per cent of all people who die do so after the age of 65 years.

Table 2.1 Deaths by cause 1979, England and Wales (selected major causes only).

Condition (International Classification of Disease)	Total	%
All causes	593 019	100.0
Neoplasms (ICD 140–239)	129 638	21.9
Diseases of the circulatory system (ICD 390–458)	298 436	50.3
Diseases of the respiratory system (ICD 460–519)	85 925	14.5
Diseases of the digestive system (ICD 520–577)	16 255	2.7
Accidents, poisonings and violence (ICD E800–E999)	21 153	3.6
Other causes	41 612	7.0

Where death occurs in the first year of life it happens most frequently before the end of the first week after birth. The main causes are immaturity, birth injury and congenital abnormalities. Thereafter until the end of the first year the most significant causes of death are, in order, chest disease, congenital abnormalities, 'sudden infant death syndrome', infectious disease and accidents, poisonings and violence.

From age 1–14 years, accidents are the commonest cause of death followed by cancer, congenital abnormalities and respiratory disease.

From 15–64 years, there are striking differences between the sexes. In men coronary heart disease is by far the most common cause, followed by lung cancer, other cancers and strokes. In women cancer is the leading cause of death with the breast being the commonest organ affected, followed by heart disease and strokes.

Trends in mortality

Deaths from many diseases for which medical treatments are available (i.e. infectious diseases) have been showing a steady downward trend and this trend was well established before the discovery of antibiotics. Notable among these has been tuberculosis. Recently there has also been a decrease in reported deaths due to hypertensive disease, cancer of the stomach, bronchitis, suicide, strokes and, in men, cancer of the lung. The rise in ischaemic heart disease seems to have levelled off and only in cancer of the lung in women is a marked upward trend still being observed. In general the average expected lifespan at birth has been steadily increasing in all developed countries. This has been mostly due to improvements in mortality in babies. However even after the age of 50 there has been a small increase in life expectancy which has made some contribution to the trend towards longevity.

Theoretical impact of future successful medical care

What theoretical effect would the elimination of certain diseases have on total population mortality? Calculations have been made which suggest that a cure for all heart disease would add 12–13 years to average life expectancy at birth and a cure for all cancers would add a further 8 years. If all known diseases were cured, the average life span would be about 100 years with all people then dying from old age. It is perhaps a sobering thought that if medicine were totally successful, its major contribution would be to add about 25 years of healthy old age.

The value of current clinical practice

However, more important than such improbable speculations about future medical advances is the observation that when death is looked at from the perspective of the community, certain important questions can be asked about the value of current clinical care and the way it influences health and survival. While some causes of death are falling because of our clinical care or because of changes in the nature of disease over time (secular trends), other causes of death, such as breast cancer and asthma, are remaining remarkably constant, despite new therapeutic advances. This could be due to a complex interaction between a rising incidence of deaths from these causes being offset by successful therapy or, more simply, due to the ineffectiveness of some therapies at preventing death.

The value of epidemiological studies, whether they are investigations carried out on generally available mortality data or carefully designed controlled trials is that they enable us to observe the usefulness of our clinical interventions.

International comparisons of mortality

Figure 2.1 shows one use of routinely collected mortality data in a comparison of deaths from 'preventable causes' in six developed countries: UK, USA, France, Japan, Italy and Sweden. The causes of death chosen for comparison included tuberculosis, cancer of the cervix, Hodgkins' disease, hypertensive disease, acute respiratory infection, pneumonia, appendicitis, thyroid imbalance, avitaminosis, chronic rheumatic heart disease, acute and chronic cholecystitis, infant mortality and maternal deaths. Reported deaths from these causes were examined over a 24 year period from 1951. The figure shows that the general trend of preventable deaths in most countries was both downward and rapid compared to the general pattern of mortality. There was also found a dramatic progression for Japan from high to low mortality from these causes over the period of the study.

In general this analysis provided evidence in support of the hypothesis that medical services can have an impact on certain disease conditions. However it is difficult to extricate the effect of medical care from other important possible influences such as different social habits and standards of living. There is a danger of overinterpretation of such analyses since comparisons are not between similar populations but between different races with different diets, social habits and genetic tendencies.

Morbidity

Morbidity is a general term given to measures of ill health. It can be assessed by examination of medical records, sickness certificates,

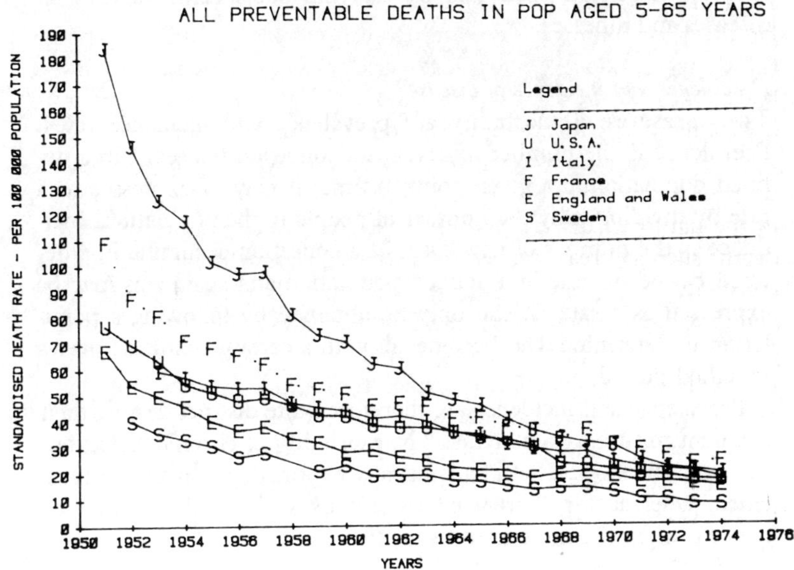

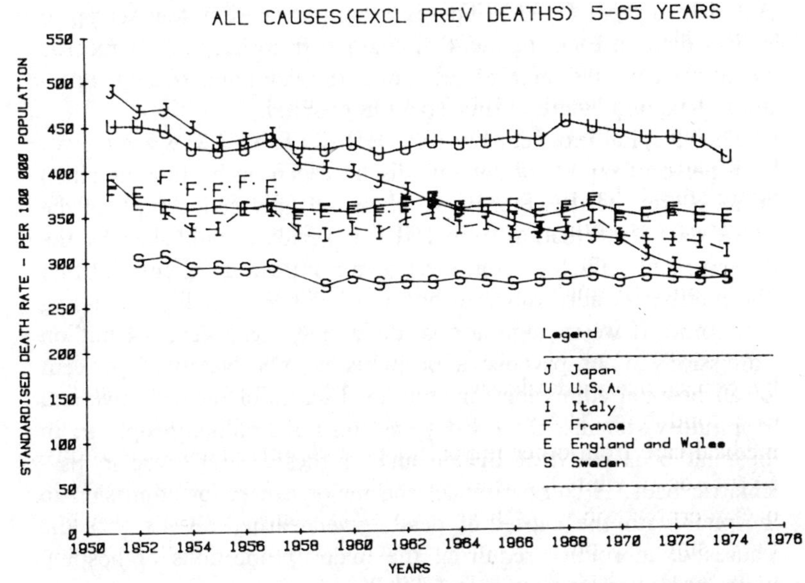

Fig. 2.1 Comparison of time trends in mortality from 'preventable causes' (see text for definition) with mortality from all causes in six countries 1951–74. The figure was kindly provided by J. Charlton.

hospital admissions data and by carrying out specific surveys on diseases and illnesses.

Prevalence and incidence of disease

Two measures of morbidity are prevalence and incidence rates. Prevalence is the number of cases of a condition that exist in a defined population at a given point in time; it may be expressed as a rate by dividing it by the number of people in the population. Incidence is the number of new cases of a condition occurring in a defined period of time in a defined population and again this may be expressed as a rate. It can only be obtained by following a population to determine who becomes ill with a certain condition over a specified period.

Prevalence and incidence are therefore quite distinct despite their frequent misuse as synonyms. The morbidity of chronic conditions such as arthritis and asthma is usually expressed in terms of prevalence, whereas for short-lived conditions such as influenza, incidence is often the more useful statistic.

Hospital admissions

In the UK there are routinely collected and published sources of data on hospital admissions. The most complete is the Hospital Activity Analysis (HAA). This is a computerised system set up to collect data on each inpatient discharged from hospital. It records details of age, sex, area of residence, the condition treated, operation data, and length of time spent in hospital.

The Hospital Inpatient Enquiry (HIPE) (Table 2.2) is a survey of a 10 per cent sample of patients discharged from hospital obtained in most areas of the country by taking a 10 per cent sample of the HAA data. Information from HIPE is regularly published by the Government (OPCS). From these sources it can be discovered that the number of admissions to hospital has been steadily increasing over time. If we exclude normal deliveries, there were 4.4 million admissions to non-psychiatric hospitals in 1978. Nearly 25 per cent of all hospital admissions are due to diseases of the digestive and respiratory systems. On any day one-third of a million people are in hospital beds in Great Britain and of these 130 000 are in psychiatric beds. A comparison of the major causes for admission to hospital with the causes of death given earlier reveals that the causes of morbidity requiring the major proportions of hospital time and resources are quite different from the major causes of mortality.

Table 2.2 Estimated total discharges and deaths from hospital (HIPE, 1978) by selected major causes.

Condition (ICD)	Estimated total	%
All causes	4 407 740	100.0
Neoplasms (ICD 140–239)	455 840	10.3
Diseases of the circulatory system (ICD 390–458)	507 570	11.5
Diseases of the respiratory system (ICD 460–519)	370 060	8.4
Diseases of the digestive system (ICD 520–577)	453 790	10.2
Accidents, poisonings and violence (ICD E800–E999)	555 260	12.6
Other causes	2 065 220	47.0

Sickness absence

After hospital admissions, the next most useful indicator of moderate morbidity is routinely collected sickness absence data from National Insurance certificates. Unfortunately these data are limited to employed people and exclude many women who do not work, all children and most pensioners. Furthermore, the patient only becomes eligible for sickness benefit after the first 3 consecutive days of illness not counting Sundays. Since mid-1982 patients have had to certify themselves as 'off sick' for their first 7 days of illness although the eligibility for benefit has remained unchanged. This change may limit the value of this data source.

Examination of the frequency of certified sickness reveals that over a million people are off sick each month, mostly with minor ailments. Sickness absence, particularly short term absence, has been steadily rising, in contrast to mortality, which has been falling.

In general, statistics relating to the causes for being off sick are unreliable because doctors may not record proper diagnoses for social or other reasons. For example, people with marital problems or depression may be recorded as having 'viral illness' or 'backache'.

General practice morbidity

General practitioners see the full range of health problems from the child with a cold to the old man dying of cancer. A series of surveys has been undertaken to examine the nature of general practice attendances. The first survey in 1955–6 covered 170 practices (General Register Office, 1958). The second in 1970–2 (OPCS, 1974; Royal College of General Practitioners, 1979) only involved 57 practices but it was continued until 1976 with 20 practices. The analyses record the number of consultations or series of consultations for a given problem tabulated by the patient's age and sex. The numbers of consultations or series of consultations for a given

Table 2.3 Estimated consultations in general practice by selected major causes. (OPCS 1970–1.)

Condition (ICD)	Rate per 1000 population	%
All causes	3009.6	100.0
Neoplasms (ICD 140–239)	44.8	1.5
Diseases of the circulatory system (ICD 390–445)	254.3	8.4
Diseases of the respiratory system (ICD 460–519)	567.8	18.9
Diseases of the digestive system (ICD 520–577)	120.8	4.0
Accidents poisonings and violence (ICD N800–N999)	159.5	5.3
Other causes	1862.4	61.9

problem are also tabulated by the patient's age, sex, diagnosis and whether the patient was referred elsewhere (Table 2.3).

The position of the GP within the health care system is unique and his approach to health problems provides the greatest argument for the value of a community perspective on the problems of ill health. Fry (1979) has analysed the diagnoses made in his own practice for over 25 years. Upper respiratory infections, emotional disorders and chronic mental illness, skin disorders, gastrointestinal disorders and rheumatism and arthritis were the commonest reasons for consultation. He also spent considerable time on preventive care.

Indeed because as much as 70 per cent of the total community may consult a GP in the course of a year and over 90 per cent in a 5 year period, the GP is in an ideal position to use his knowledge of the community to promote preventive measures.

For example, he might use the opportunity of the consultation to take his patient's blood pressure to detect hypertension even though investigation of the presenting problem may not call for this. Such action is termed 'case-finding' and is based on the recognition that certain risk factors for disease can be present without the knowledge of the patient but which once detected and controlled could improve the outlook for his future health.

Illness

The symptom is the last measure of morbidity to be considered. Morrell (1972) has investigated the common symptoms, such as cough and headache, which patients present to doctors for further advice. Obviously a proportion of symptoms are due to definable serious disease but he found that many symptoms are due to minor conditions which are self-limiting. This means that simply waiting, with or without drugs to give relief, results in their resolution. That

Table 2.4 Number of consultations per 1000 patients at risk for 14 common symptoms, by sex. (From: Morrell, 1972.)

Condition	Males	Females
Cough	240	287
Rashes	127	165
Pain in throat	125	162
Adbominal pain	95	102
Disturbance of bowel function	92	93
Spots, sores and ulcers	78	103
Back pain	82	90
Chest pain	83	85
Headache	70	79
Joint pain	66	75
Disturbance of gastric function	61	80
Changes in balance	22	43
Disturbance of breathing	30	29
Changes of energy	15	43

many symptoms are handled by personal stoicism, friendly lay advice or pharmacists is very important to the efficient running of a health service. It is certain that the health care services would be totally overwhelmed if everyone took every symptom to the doctor. The scale and distribution of symptoms taken to GPs is shown in Table 2.4.

From examination of Tables 2.1–2.4 it can be seen that the principal underlying causes of death are diseases of the circulatory system, neoplasm and respiratory disease, accidents, poisonings and violence and finally diseases of the digestive system. These causes account for 93 per cent of all deaths. However they are only responsible for 53 per cent of hospital discharges and 38.1 per cent of general practice attendances.

It can also be seen that neoplasms are an important cause of death and hospital admission but are a relatively rare cause of GP consultation. Certain conditions, notably psychiatric illness, account for much more morbidity than mortality, whereas respiratory disease is an equally important cause of both mortality and morbidity.

FACTORS INFLUENCING MORTALITY AND MORBIDITY

One of the essential features of community medicine is the search for the determinants of ill health. These may be divided into intrinsic causes such as genetic factors and extrinsic causes such as pollutants, infections, and lifestyle habits such as smoking.

Intrinsic determinants of disease

Population changes and ill health

In the preceeding description of health problems, the important part played by ageing has already been discussed. There are, however, many other demographic characteristics that profoundly influence the nature and distribution of disease. These include sex, social class distribution and ethnic origins. Such a total view of the population as the substrate upon which diseases flourish or perish provides us with a framework on which the likely causes of morbidity and mortality can be considered.

Age distribution

The total population of the UK has increased by almost 50 per cent since the beginning of the twentieth century. The proportion of the population above retirement age (60 years for women and 65 years for men) was only 6 per cent in 1901, but by 1981 it had risen to 16 per cent. This change has had a profound impact on the distribution and frequency of diseases, particularly chronic degenerative disorders and neoplasms. It is also relevant to the structure of the community particularly in relation to the availability of younger people to care for the sick and the elderly.

There are now 5.2 million men and women aged 65–74 in the UK and a further 3.2 million who are over 75. Over 90 per cent of these elderly people are able to live in their own homes. Where necessary they are supported by home helps, meals on wheels, district nurses, health visitors, general practitioners and voluntary organisations, but most look after themselves or are cared for by friends or relatives. It is estimated that the number of those over 75 years will increase by nearly one-third before the turn of the century.

An increasing number of elderly people will result in an increase in the number of disabled. Clinically the young rarely have more than one organ system affected by disease but in the elderly multiple pathology is common. This can complicate patient care, since what might be good management for one problem may be bad for another.

There are some problems of the elderly which illustrate how increasing age affects health. It has been estimated, for example, that 25 per cent of all people over 65 years have hearing difficulties. It would appear that in noisy urban industrial environments auditory function is particularly liable to deterioration over time. Although hearing aids are readily available and have been supplied to over one million people, the elderly are frequently reluctant either to use the aids they have or to ask for aids when they need them. They may be embarrassed by being seen wearing an aid, which may be considered a stigma.

Another example is blindness in the elderly. This is chiefly due to senile degeneration, cataract formation, glaucoma and diabetes and is much more socially disabling than deafness. Over 14 000 new cases of blindness are registered in the UK each year and most of these are elderly. The careful management of glaucoma and diabetes may prevent loss of sight and cataract surgery can restore vision. There are however many parts of the world where such surgical facilities are not readily available and where additional causes of visual loss are prevalent such as trachoma.

Loss of mobility is a further common problem amongst the elderly. This is usually due to osteoarthritis, the sequelae of stroke or hip injury, although occasionally less serious foot problems such as bunions or corns may be significant factors in preventing an elderly person from walking.

All these disabilities particularly when associated with cerebral atherosclerosis may result in social isolation and depression. Often the price of longevity is to outlast one's relatives and friends and this may also be associated with dietary neglect and increased risk of accident and injury. Perhaps worst of all is the danger that elderly people with perfectly normal cerebral faculties will be patronised and categorised as senile and thus allocated to less than adequate geriatric medical facilities alongside demented contemporaries with whom they can have little contact.

Social class

Like old age, low social class is associated with increased mortality and morbidity. This is true for nearly every condition with the exception of breast cancer. Why social class should be quite such an important factor in health is, however, far from clear.

The observation that some jobs are more hazardous than others cannot be the explanation, since the effect of social class is equally well observed in wives whose exposure to work-related risk factors is completely different, yet they are classified into the same social class as their husbands. Furthermore, the ability of an individual to change jobs means that social classification itself is not a fixed personal characteristic. It may be, however, that the healthy are more likely to rise in social class and the sick to fall which may provide some partial explanation of the health differences observed between classes.

Parity

Despite the rise in population size there has been paradoxically a dramatic decline in the numbers of births and overall family size assisted by new developments in the field of contraception and abortion. Recently there have been fewer older women giving birth. As a result, the number of children diagnosed as having Down's syndrome, a condition known to be common in children born to older women, has decreased by over one-quarter during the last 25 years. The recent availability of amniocentesis karyotype screening and genetic counselling may further accelerate the decline in the number of children surviving with the syndrome.

Genetic factors

Many common conditions have a genetic or familial basis and detailed accounts of these are available in other textbooks (e.g. Cavalli-Sforza & Bodmer, 1978). The study of families and communities is often the means by which genetic cause is confirmed. The expression of genetic tendencies may well require the appropriate stimulus from the environment. It is, however, very difficult to ascertain how much of the aetiology of the problem may be due to environmental and hence potentially preventable causes and how much is of irremediable genetic origin. In asthma, for example, it seems likely that in some cases the illness only expresses itself in the presence of suitable environmental trigger factors, such as allergies, whereas in other cases no environmental factor appears to operate. The knowledge that certain conditions such as hypertension run in families can be used to identify populations at risk and thus facilitate preventive health measures (Heller et al, 1980).

Immigration

The other important change that has influenced health is migration. People move in pursuit of employment both within and outside their country of birth. Such social uprooting may have an effect on health. Often immigrant people start to develop the diseases of their adopted country. This is particularly true when life style and diet is changed.

There are marked differences in the way people from various immigrant subcultures view their illnesses and in the way they use health services. Also there are certain diseases such as tuberculosis and rickets that are still common in their countries of origin, which immigrants may import with them.

Language difficulties, particularly amongst women who may rarely leave the home, and educational deficiencies make health information difficult to transmit. Differences in the ways in which immigrants view the status of women and of teenagers may produce great strains in families who have to live with the constant comparison of the customs of their adopted country.

EXTRINSIC DETERMINANTS OF DISEASE

Life habits and health

Just as the role of bacteria was discovered to be important in the aetiology of so much disease in the nineteenth century, evidence has been accumulating of the importance of certain harmful life habits as a cause of ill health through the twentieth century. The ways in which eating and exercise habits influence health are difficult to unravel. Certainly the inhalation of noxious substances such as cigarette smoke and solvents have psychological as well as physical consequences. Similarly overindulgence in food and abuse of alcohol have similar effects. However, although lack of exercise may result in loss of fitness, the evidence that it actually causes disease is not very convincing. The phenomenon of fit young men dropping dead with myocardial infarction is well recognised and is a good illustration of the difference between fitness and health.

Cigarette smoking

The importance of smoking as a risk factor for disease is considerable: coronary heart disease, lung cancer, chronic bronchitis and peripheral vascular disease are all significantly more common in smokers. Babies born to smoking mothers have a lower birth weight with the attendant increase in perinatal health hazards. There has been a gradual decline in smoking in men and in the professional classes in recent years. However, there has been a slight rise in the proportion of women smoking and men who continue to smoke are consuming more cigarettes per head.

Alcoholism

The chronic ingestion of alcohol in amounts equivalent to more than 3 pints of beer a day can cause damage to a variety of organs, chiefly the brain and liver. Obesity and hypertension are frequent sequelae of heavy drinking. However evidence from several major studies suggests that modest regular drinking as opposed to alcohol abuse may actually protect health. This may possibly be related to the association between alcohol intake and increases in the levels of high density lipoproteins (HDL) which are thought to reduce atheroma. Some ethnic groups seem particularly prone to alcoholism whereas others rarely suffer from it. This suggests that cultural and genetic factors are important in this problem.

Drug abuse

The abuse of drugs is conventionally divided into three categories: the abuse of medically prescribed drugs, such as tranquillisers; the abuse of soft illicit drugs such as cannabis resin; and the abuse of hard drugs, such as heroin.

Each of these forms of abuse are viewed differently by society and they have very different social effects.

There were 50 million prescriptions issued for psychoactive drugs in 1980. The chief hazard of such prescriptions apart from the sedation of machine operators is that of providing the instrument for self destruction.

The abuse of cannabis has received much attention not least because of the campaign to legalise it. Certainly, apart from mild bronchitis in heavy users, the medical effects of abusing this drug seem minimal. The same cannot be said for other soft drugs such as amphetamine which in addition to causing acute psychosis in overdose may also result in domestic and social violence that may pose as many social difficulties as the abuse of hard drugs such as opiates, LSD, and cocaine.

The abuse of hard drugs may produce disastrous health and social effects. Death from septicaemia is a major hazard amongst those injecting the drug intravenously. The social problems of prostitution and theft are the almost invariable accompaniment of opiate abuse because of the enormous cost of maintaining the habit. However, some addicts achieve a relatively successful accommodation with their drugs and although the natural history of drug abuse is inadequately understood, many opiate addicts are known to abandon their habits spontaneously as they reach middle age. However, during the 1970s the number of notified addicts of both sexes receiving treatment has nearly doubled.

Diet

There has been a gradual change in diet in many developed countries. Affluence has resulted in the greater consumption of sugar and other carbohydrates causing an increased prevalence of obesity, dental decay and diabetes. How food may cause other diseases has also been intensively studied. The role of animal fats in causing coronary artery disease is still questionable. Food allergies are currently popularly considered to be at the root of many common ailments. The hard scientific evidence for this is however scanty, although there seems no doubt that asthma, rhinitis and eczema can be due to allergies to foods such as cows' milk.

Changes in sexual mores

In recent times there has been a change in public attitudes towards sexual behaviour. Divorce has become more common and more couples are living together without marriage. Contraception, particularly by the contraceptive pill, is now widely accepted by society. All these changes have produced marked medical and social effects. Venereal infection has remained prevalent despite the availability of antibiotics (although in the last few years its incidence has decreased). Marital relationships have become subject to greater strains and broken families are now commonplace with greater risks of emotional upset to growing children and psychological stress to their parents. Young girls, in particular, are highly liable to suffer depressive illness in adulthood if subjected to emotional disturbances, such as their parents divorcing around the time of menarche. Expectations from relationships have changed considerably and both men and women have become more confused about their roles within marriage and society. Movements such as Women's Lib have tended to highlight the profound social change of women's progress towards equal social status in society. In developed countries the working wife and mother is becoming more common than the housewife and this makes for greater difficulties in child rearing and in creating cohesiveness in the local community.

The use of leisure time

Two major changes in the use of leisure time affect health: mechanical transport has decreased the necessity to walk and television watching has become the major activity in most adult lives, apart from sleeping and working. Evidence has gradually been accumulating to show that inactivity during work and leisure time is a risk factor for mortality in general, although its relation to ischaemic heart disease seems to be less strong than for the major risk factors for the disease (Salonen et al, 1982).

The physical environment at work and home

Modern industry produces a variety of pollutants that may be dangerous to health including the noise often associated with manufacturing processes. Legislation has sought to cut the more harmful emissions of smoke, chemicals and radiation but such pollution control frequently conflicts with commercial interests and may even make certain manufacturing processes uneconomic. In some situations people may even have to choose between their health and having employment. The ways in which smoke and other air pollutants can be hazardous in the home are also of great importance. Fires, accidental poisonings and accidents are often attributable to inadequate safety precautions in the home. Similarly accidents at work are frequently found to be caused by failure to take precautions.

RISKS AND ASSETS

A general view of the risk of disease

The term 'at risk' is attributable to the whole of one group relative to another. The individuals in the group said to be at risk are not all necessarily ill or diseased but simply more likely in the future to develop problems. This is most easily illustrated by the wearing of safety belts in cars. People who do not wear them are known to be more likely to be injured in an accident than those who do. However it is obvious that if someone chooses not to wear a seat belt he will not necessarily have an accident.

Asset factors

Recently it has been recognised that there are definable characteristics in a population which are the opposite of risk factors. These have been called 'assets' or asset factors. Nuckolls et al (1972) showed in a study of women having babies, that the social assets of a supportive network of family and friends protected those experiencing stresses around the time of childbirth from a variety of diseases. Also the observation that widowers have a significantly higher predicted mortality from all causes may be evidence that having a wife is a social asset protective to health. How important asset factors are or how they may be used to prevent disease is still uncertain.

CONCLUSION

The study of the whole community in search of the causes of health problems and their solution is a rewarding and important part of medicine. The complex interaction of many factors, some preventing and others causing disease can be readily observed to operate both within communities and individuals. For most conditions our ignorance of cause is still profound but the vantage point of community medicine has often proved useful. Two hundred years ago, the country practitioner Jenner asked one of his elderly patients why she thought milkmaids never caught smallpox and was told all about cowpox. He had been looking at the healthy and asking why. This single observation has resulted in the global eradication of smallpox because the factor that had determined the health of milkmaids could be transferred to everyone else. The methods of community medicine are naturally focused on the prevention of disease and when successful their benefits can be immense.

REFERENCES

Cavalli-Sforza L L, Bodmer W F 1978 The genetics of human populations. Freeman, San Francisco

Department of Health and Social Security. Health and personal social services statistics for England. HMSO, London. Published annually

Department of Health and Social Security, Office of Population Censuses and Surveys, Welsh Office. Hospital In-patient Enquiry, England and Wales. HMSO, London. Published annually

Fry J 1979 Common diseases: their nature incidence and care. MTP Press Ltd, Lancaster

General Register Office 1958 Studies in medical and population subjects No 14. Morbidity statistics from general practice 1955–56 (Vols I–III). HMSO, London

Heller R F, Robinson N, Peart W S 1980 Value of blood-pressure measurement in relatives of hypertensive patients. Lancet i:1206–8

Morrell D C 1972 Symptom interpretation in general practice. Journal of the Royal College of General Practitioners 22: 297–309

Nuckolls K B, Cassel J, Kaplan B H 1972 Psychosocial assets, life crisis and the prognosis of pregnancy. American Journal of Epidemiology 95: 431–41

Office of Population Censuses and Surveys 1974 Studies on medical and population subjects No 26. Morbidity statistics from general practice. Second national study 1970–1. HMSO, London

Royal College of General Practitioners, Office of Population Censuses and Surveys, Department of Health and Social Security 1979. Studies on medical and population subjects No 36. Morbidity statistics from general practice 1971–2. Second national study. HMSO, London

Salonen J T, Puska P, Tuomilehto J 1982 Physical activity and risk of myocardial infarction, cerebral stroke and death. American Journal of Epidemiology 115: 526–37

3

The epidemiological approach

The investigation of disease patterns and their changes over time requires some measure of the number of healthy and ill people in the community. Simple analyses may need no more than the calculation of prevalence or incidence rates based on a numerator of affected people and a denominator of all the people in a defined group. More sophisticated analyses for determining the aetiology of disease extend the data from head counts to measurements of each person's relevant attributes such as height, blood pressure or disability and of the environment with which he comes into contact.

A variety of methods has been developed over the years for the investigation of epidemiological and health service problems. In this chapter we describe some of the these methods and give examples of how these methods are used to answer epidemiological questions. The use of routinely collected data on mortality, often the first step in the analysis of a problem, is discussed, followed by consideration of how studies may be designed to answer specific hypotheses about cause and effect. Some of the examples come from the study of air pollution, so the scene is set by a short history of the subject. The political repercussions of the epidemiological studies of air pollution are discussed in Chapter 7.

AIR POLLUTION AND ITS RISE TO INFAMY

The study of the effects on health of air polluted with smoke and the consequences of the reduction in domestic and industrial emissions is one of a small number of examples in which the whole process of observation, epidemiological research and successful action can be found. This is used here to illustrate the way in which ideas grow and epidemiological research is done and, at the same time, to act as a framework for some of the underlying theory.

Air pollution has been a problem for many years. In 1257, Henry III's Queen Eleanor is reputed to have left Nottingham because of the smoke, never to return. In 1273, an Act of Parliament was passed forbidding the burning of coal in London, for which offence in 1306 a man was executed. John Evelyn, the seventeenth century diarist, wrote a complete treatise describing the outpouring of smoke from local industry near St James and its effect on buildings, lifestyle and health. Although of some interest to Charles II, who not only wished to improve the quality of life in London, but may have been concerned for his own health, the treatise was not followed by remedial action. The Industrial Revolution brought further pollution to the air, both from coal which fuelled the factories and from the domestic hearth. There were episodes of smog in London in the last quarter of the nineteenth century, 5 of which together have been estimated to have caused 4750 deaths.

The London smog of 1952

London used to be renowned for its pea-soupers, limiting vision to less than the width of a road junction. The worst recorded episode occurred from December 5–8, 1952. Once the damage was realised it became the major stimulus to modern epidemiological research into air pollution, but at the time, probably because familiarity with smog had left the authorities unwary, no steps were taken to protect the public. The first suspicion of a disaster was raised when several prize animals at the Smithfield Agricultural Show either died or had to be slaughtered—an example of biological monitoring on the grand scale. The medical profession was made aware of the impact on human health when it was found that florists had run out of flowers. No official warning was given: a news item which was to be broadcast on the last day of the smog advising of possible dangers was withdrawn and the press failed to appreciate the threat of the smog to public health. It was some days after the smog when The Times reported on December 20 that it had been announced in the House of Commons that during the week ending December 13, 4703 deaths had occurred in Greater London compared with 1852 in the same week in 1951.

Two papers appeared in *The Lancet* in January, 1953, describing the effects of the smog on the demand for medical care. The Emergency Bed Service, an organisation which keeps account of beds available for emergency admissions in London hospitals, provided evidence of an immediate increase in morbidity from the smog by the rapid increase in requests for beds from the first day of the smog. Cheek by jowl in the same issue was a paper on the greatly increased number of attendances at one general practice for respiratory disorders consequent to the smog.

The most impressive evidence, however, came from an analysis of mortality returns carried out by W.P.D. Logan, Chief Medical Statistician in the General Register Office, and reported in *The Lancet* of February 14, 1953. The paper is worth reviewing in a little detail to bring out some of the ways in which mortality data may be used to draw a picture of events. Logan justified the analysis by pointing out the enormity of the effects of the London smog when compared with two other famous episodes, one in the Meuse Valley in 1930, which caused 64 deaths, and the other in the Pennsylvania mining town of Donora in 1948 from which 20 deaths occurred. The events in London were two orders of magnitude greater.

Logan first compared the number of deaths by week in 1952 with the average weekly number in the years 1947–52. In the 2 weeks straddled by the smog there were almost exactly 3000 more deaths in 1952 than in the previous years and a further 1000 extra deaths occurred in the following week. Excess deaths were also observed in each week thereafter, though Logan felt these might have been due to factors other than the smog since there was already a small number of excess deaths recorded in the week before the smog.

Having established that a departure from the expected mortality followed the smog for the whole of the Greater London population of 8.5 million, Logan divided the mortality figures according to the geographic boundaries of administrative areas: the inner London Administrative County, the outer ring of Greater London and the 160 great towns of England and Wales excluding London. Despite the presence of dense fog in some of the great towns, their mortality record for the weeks ending November 29 to January 10 suggested no more than 164 excess deaths could be associated with the period of the London smog. The outer ring of Greater London in aggregate showed a proportional increase in mortality not much below that for inner London.

The London data were then divided by age at death. Although the deaths were few in number in the age range 0–1 year, the number doubled (from 28 to 54) from the week ending December 6 to the week ending December 13. There were increases in mortality from ages 1–44 years of about 50 per cent, but over age 44 mortality in the week of the smog was nearly 300 per cent more than in the previous week (it is commonly said that only the very young and the elderly suffered from the smog, but this statement depends heavily on the definition of elderly!)

Causes of death written on death certificates are renowned for their limited accuracy, particularly in the absence of post-mortem data; they suffer from misdiagnosis even within the major rubrics of the International Classification of Diseases. However, assuming that the population including the doctors were probably not aware of the effects of the smog, it would seem that all diagnoses should increase at a time of increased mortality if the signing physicians were not biased by circumstances. *A priori* the effects of the smog should have been to increase mortality from respiratory and cardiovascular disease. Within the London Administrative County mortality from bronchitis increased eight times and that from pneumonia three times. Deaths from cancer of the lung, coronary disease, myocardial degeneration and 'other respiratory diseases' also increased whereas deaths from suicide were unchanged. Deaths from motor vehicle accidents were also unchanged, probably because the increased risk of an accident due to reduced visibility was balanced by the reduced risk due to lower speeds and a smaller number of vehicles on the road.

Finally, an analysis of the number of daily deaths from December 1–15, showed an increase in deaths even on December 5, the first day of the smog, in comparison with the four preceding days and the increase was still evident on December 15, the last day in the analysis.

Logan ended his discussion expressing the hope that such an event would never be allowed to recur. The political reaction to the mortality from the smog is taken up in Chapter 7 where the policies derived from the epidemiological data are examined.

PROBLEM SOLVING IN EPIDEMIOLOGY

Posing the question

Some basic concept of causation or interrelation is needed before a problem can be analysed. The classic model is a triangular one of association between the host, the agent and the environment. This is suitable to a large extent for infectious diseases, where the agent is of crucial importance, but is inadequate for chronic degenerative diseases when there may be many agents all of which could be seen as part of the environment and which react with the host. A more useful model treats the host as a genetic central core on which the environment acts through biological, social and physical effects to produce dysfunction. This allows the single cause concept implied in the classic model but emphasises the contribution of multiple factors to disease causation. It may be written in a semi-mathematical form:

$$\text{Health status} = \text{person} + \text{place} + \text{time},$$

which is convenient when we want to convert hypotheses into a statistically testable format. Personal factors include demographic variables such as marital status, social class and ethnic group; biological attributes such as serum cholesterol levels, obesity or blood group and socially determined attributes such as attitudes towards immunisation or support networks. Geographic factors include measures of the environment related to place. The effects on health status of changes in the personal and geographic factors may be assessed from trends over time, the third term in the equation.

In Logan's study of mortality, the model related two principal factors to each other, mortality and the day of the month, the latter as a proxy for level of pollution (not very accurate, though a clever device when he had no other data to hand). He looked at other factors which might have influenced the relation he observed between the principal factors, including age and location. The evidence from age and location helped to explain some of the variation in mortality which might otherwise have been erroneously attributed to the smog. He also used cause-specific mortality to refine his measure of outcome, thereby excluding causes of mortality unlikely to be attributable to the smog.

Mortality studies

There have been many mortality studies since 1953, some on the events of 1952, some on similar episodes in other cities and some on the effects of pollution over whole countries. Acute events such as a smog could be quantified after a fashion using data other than precise measures of the pollutants in the air because indisputable qualitative differences existed from one time to another. To estimate the health effects of pollution over more subtle variations in concentration, measures to differentiate between the levels were needed. An ingenious method was devised by Charles Daly (1959) in the 1950s when there were very few pollution monitoring stations in the UK. He wanted to find out whether mortality in the county boroughs of England and Wales varied with pollution levels. During the Second World War records were kept of the distribution of fuel throughout the country and collection of data continued until 1952. Daly created a fuel consumption index assuming that the degree of smoke pollution, particularly from domestic sources, would be correlated with the use of coal, coke and anthracite.

In his analysis he related his index to mortality in the county boroughs from a variety of causes in the period 1948–54 (centred around the census year of 1951), taking into account the differences in social class, crowding and education between the boroughs. He found, among other things, that the death rates in middle-aged men for chronic bronchitis and malignant neoplasms of the lungs and bronchi were positively related to his pollution index. The same relations were found by Gardner and co-workers (1969) using data for the period 1958–64. At this time the effects on health resulting from the Clean Air Act of 1956 were insufficient to be detected in changes in mortality patterns.

During the late 1950s and '60s a national network of instruments was developed to measure smoke and sulphur dioxide. Data from this network were related to mortality in the county and London boroughs for the period 1969–73 and differences in many socio-economic and climatic variables which might have influenced the results were taken into account (Chinn et al, 1981). In these analyses no association was found between mortality from chronic bronchitis or neoplasms of the lungs and bronchi and either contemporary levels of smoke and sulphur dioxide or Daly's 20-year-old index. This series of studies which considered cross-sections of mortality at different periods and related each new finding with what had been found before, suggests that as atmospheric smoke and sulphur dioxide levels have declined so has their effect on mortality to the extent that the relation is now no longer detectable.

Ad hoc studies

The availability of routinely collected data, particularly of those that are published and easily found (see Ch. 2), makes studies such as those described above relatively easy and cheap. However the quality of the data and its suitability for any particular purpose may not be adequate either for testing hypotheses or even for describing the situation. It is often necessary to carry out *ad hoc* studies to collect information specific to the problem in hand.

Descriptive studies

Epidemiological studies make use of natural rather than designed experiments as it may be both impractical and unethical to deliberately expose healthy people to factors believed to be causally associated with disease. Several methods have been developed to take advantage of naturally occurring contrasts in exposure. The simplest approach is descriptive and is similar to what we have already seen. It consists of counting biological events such as death, cases of influenza or number of diabetics in a community which may then be analysed according to other host characteristics such as age and sex, or related to environmental factors.

Descriptive statistics can be calculated, such as the percentage of the population with a condition or using particular health services. These may be helpful when tracing the course of an epidemic, as they may indicate the source of infection, or they may be useful in guiding decisions on where a new clinic should be sited. No hypothesis is tested, although the data may suggest hypotheses for testing in other studies.

Analytical studies

A somewhat more complex approach is that of analytical studies. These studies are often prompted by ideas or hypotheses formulated from previous experience but they may themselves be used to generate hypotheses. There are four general designs: the cross-sectional, the cohort (or longitudinal), the case-control and the randomised controlled trial (RCT). The RCT (more fully described in Ch. 4) is an experimental design in which a group of people is randomly divided into two parts, one composed of people to be exposed to a new treatment believed to be beneficial (or at least not harmful) and the other of people receiving either the conventional or an inactive (placebo) treatment. The morbidity and mortality experiences of the two groups are compared after a period of time has elapsed. The RCT is clearly unacceptable for testing factors at levels which are believed to have irreversible adverse effects on health. The three other designs are used to investigate adverse effects of inadvertent, accidental or natural exposure to supposed risk factors.

1. Cross-sectional studies

The events of December 1952 spurred a considerable amount of research in the UK to determine not only whether very high concentrations of atmospheric pollutants had serious acute effects but also the consequences of prolonged exposure to much lower levels. Many of these studies were cross-sectional in which selected attributes of a population were measured at one point in time. The data were used descriptively and prevalence rates for various conditions, frequently of the respiratory system, were calculated. The cross-sectional design can, however, be used analytically when the results are compared between two or more populations investigated by identical methods but living in areas with contrasting levels of the hazard of interest.

Sheffield study. Such a set of studies was carried out in Sheffield schoolchildren living in four areas of the city with differing ambient levels of smoke and sulphur dioxide (Lunn et al, 1967). These focused on children in their first year at primary school who on average were about 5½ years old. The study of children as young as this meant that smoking habits and occupational exposures, complicating factors in studies of adults, could be disregarded. Moreover the likelihood of their having changed residential area would be much less than for adults. Thus the authors assumed that the great majority of the children they examined had been exposed to more or less the same ambient air pollution throughout their lives. Information about the children's health and socio-economic background was obtained from their parents. The children were examined physically and asked to perform a lung function test. Information about levels of smoke and sulphur dioxide in the air came from daily recordings made by air samplers at or near the schools. The levels of smoke in the most polluted area were 3½ times those in the 'clean area' and the levels of sulphur dioxide were about 3 times higher.

Age and social class are two important demographic factors found to be associated with respiratory illness and symptoms in children. In this study there was little variation in age so its effect was ignored, but there were differences in the distribution of social class in each area which might have accounted for the differences in prevalence of symptoms between the areas. For example, the prevalence of persistent or frequent cough was 15.6 per cent in children from social class I families whereas it was 32.4 per cent in children from social class IV and V families. In the most polluted area there were proportionately nearly twice as many children from social class IV and V than in the 'clean' area. This weighting of the population of the most polluted area toward those who have more respiratory disease would tend to raise the overall prevalence of persistent cough on account of social class factors. This bias in the data may be reduced or avoided by comparing symptom frequency in different areas among children of the same social class or by making numerical adjustments to the observed prevalence rates which allow for differences in social class distribution.

In this study the former was done and a definite increase in prevalence of persistent cough with increasing levels of air pollution was seen in each of the three social class groups I + II, III, and IV + V.

In analytical cross-sectional studies one can investigate interrelations between variables and these may be taken into account when comparing prevalence estimates between populations. The hypothesis tested may imply a cause and effect relation but the design does not permit a clear cut statement; the best that can be said is that the results are consistent with a cause and effect relation. However, it is possible in a cross-sectional study to collect data about past experiences which may be used to test hypotheses as described later under case-control studies.

2. Cohort studies

The two remaining designs are used to help in elucidating the cause and effect relation. The cohort study is intuitively appropriate for looking at cause and effect. A cohort is a group of people defined at some point in time by certain characteristics such as age, sex, ethnicity, geographic location and so on. Cohorts are frequently defined by date of birth. The aim of this design is to determine whether characteristics observed at the start or appearing during the course of the study are related to later events in the health of the members of the cohort. At the start of the study, the cohort may consist only of apparently healthy people, selected by the results of an examination. Alternatively it may consist of both sick and healthy so that the progress of illness may be followed from various points in its natural history.

Berlin studies, USA. A cohort study to examine, among other things, the possible effects of air pollution on symptoms from respiratory disease and on lung function, was carried out in Berlin, an industrial town in the north of New Hampshire in the north-east of the United States (Ferris et al, 1973).

The main source of air pollution in Berlin was a Kraft pulp mill in the centre of the town which emitted sulphur compounds. Other plants producing sulphur compounds and other pollutants were operating at the beginning of the study in 1961 but, shortly after, they were closed down whereas the Kraft mill doubled in capacity.

A sample of the population in 1961 was taken of those aged 25–74 years. The respondents were given lung function tests and asked a standard set of questions about respiratory illness and associated factors such as cigarette smoking. A definition of chronic nonspecific respiratory disease was used which included chronic bronchitis diagnosed from duration of phlegm production, asthma reported to have been diagnosed previously and still present, and chronic lung disease diagnosed from positive answers to certain questions on respiratory symptoms in conjunction with reduced lung function.

In 1967 a second random sample of people was selected as well as all those people seen in 1961 who were willing to participate again (the follow-up group). Thus the results of the two prevalence studies done in 1961 and 1967 could be compared and incidence rates could be calculated for the follow-up group. The same prevalence sampling technique was used in 1973 in a third study.

The key finding was that the prevalence of chronic non-specific respiratory disease was lower in 1967 than in 1961 whereas there were no changes from 1967–73.

In the analysis of those who were followed up from 1961–7 two types of incidence rate were calculated: the attack rate, which was the percentage of people without respiratory symptoms in 1961 who had developed symptoms by 1967, and the remission rate, which was the percentage of people with symptoms in 1961 who no longer reported them in 1967. Table 3.1 shows these rates for men according to their 1967 cigarette consumption. The remission rates were substantially higher than the attack rates for all groups smoking less than 15 cigarettes a day, most noticeably for non-smokers.

Because the respondents were their own controls and the authors could find no other reason for the change in disease rates, it was suggested that the change was a reflection of the change in air pollution. No regular decline in sulphur pollution was seen over the period but total suspended particulates dropped from an average of 180 $\mu g/m^3$ in the months of August and September, 1961, to 131 $\mu g/m^3$ in 1966–7 and 80 $\mu g/m^3$ in 1973.

Unfortunately, even this result was not conclusive because other unmeasured changes in the environment may have been the cause of the improvement. Nevertheless the evidence from the cohort is more compelling than that obtained from the cross-sectional studies because the change in air pollution levels was accompanied by the hypothesised change in symptoms observed in the same people.

Chronic bronchitis. Another well known study of incidence, by Fletcher and his co-workers (1976), has changed our understanding of the natural history of chronic bronchitis. Chronic bronchitis has been an important cause of morbidity and mortality since industrialisation in Europe, affecting men about three times as often as women. In 1968, the UK death rate under this heading was 87.9 per 100 000 for men aged 35–64, accounting for 6.2 per cent of

Table 3.1 Attack and remission rates for respiratory symptoms according to cigarette smoking between 1961–7 in men aged 25–74 years. Berlin, New Hampshire, USA (From: Ferris et al, 1973.)

Cigarette consumption 1967	Number without symptoms in 1961	Attack rate (%)	Number with symptoms in 1961	Remission rate (%)
Never smoked	60	8.3	15	60.0
Ex-smoker	84	14.3	40	42.5
1–14/day	19	15.8	11	36.4
15–24/day	40	35.0	21	28.6
25 + /day	39	28.0	42	26.2

mortality in this age group, and in 1978, though less, was still 29.6 per 100 000.

Two major hypotheses for the evolution of chronic bronchitis arose from clinical, pathological and epidemiological observations. The British hypothesis stated that the first stage of chronic bronchitis was mucus hypersecretion due to cigarette smoking, air pollution or infections. The mucus reduced the resistance of the bronchial tree to infections which in turn gave rise to bronchial obstruction and emphysema. The corollary was that chronic bronchitis could be prevented as soon as a persistent cough occurred by removing the stimulus and by the use of chemotherapy.

An alternative 'Dutch hypothesis' suggested that the components of chronic non-specific lung disease, namely chronic bronchitis, emphysema and asthma, were closely linked. Airway narrowing occurred in people reactive to various environmental stimuli. The narrowed airways were then more susceptible to infection, but infection was not seen as the main precursor to obstruction. If this hypothesis were correct then removal of the allergen or external stimulus would be of major importance in preventing progression of the disease and the treatment of infection would be a minor consideration.

To test these hypotheses and to determine more clearly what the natural history of chronic bronchitis was, Fletcher and his colleagues started a long-term cohort study in 1961. They planned to follow a large number of men (because chronic bronchitis is much more common in men than women) over a period of years by examining them every 6 months.

For a study lasting 8 years it was important that the cohort was made up of people unlikely to move to another part of the country or further, and thus out of reach of the researchers. Men working in London Transport Workshops and the Post Office in the northwest of London were chosen because of their known stability of residence. A preliminary questionnaire survey was carried out to find who had chronic respiratory symptoms.

Just over 3000 men aged 30–59 were questioned. As this number was too large for further investigation, a sample of 1000 of them was selected at different sampling rates from four groups according to whether (1) they had chronic phlegm production or recent chest illness (the symptomatic group), or (2) were asymptomatic nonsmokers or (3) asymptomatic smokers and ex-smokers or (4) had not returned the questionnaire. Of the 1136 men finally selected 792 remained in the study for 8 years.

Every 6 months the men were asked questions about their chest

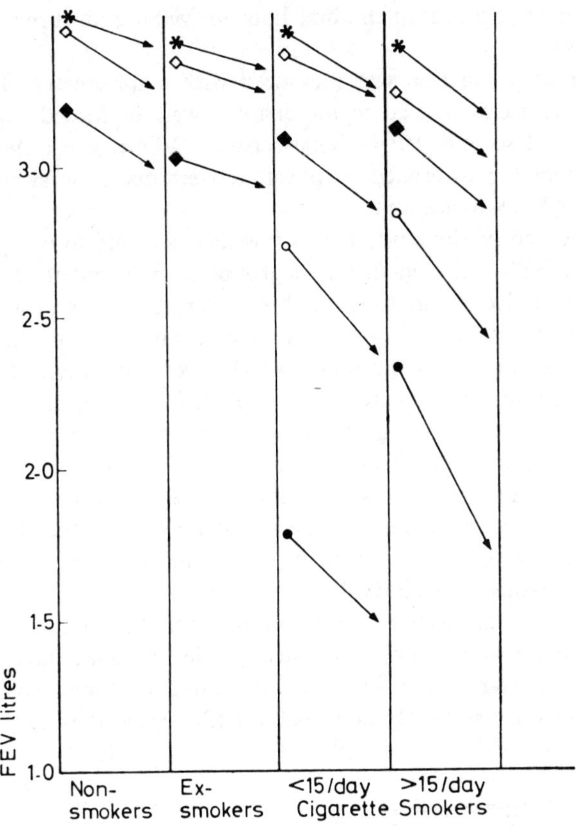

* over 80 %

◇ 75-80 %

◆ 65-75 %

○ 55-65 %

• < 55 %

Fig. 3.1 Rate of decline of FEV according to FEV/VC and smoking habits in men. The sign at the left hand end of each arrow indicates the initial mean FEV/VC of the group (given as a % in the legend) and the slope of the line indicates the mean decline over 7 years. (From: Fletcher C M et al 1970 In: Orie N, van der Lende (eds) Bronchitis III. Royal Vangorcum, Assen, p114. Reproduced with permission from the authors and the publisher.)

illnesses and about the quantity and prevalence of their phlegm. They were also asked to bring in for measurement the phlegm they had coughed up during the first hour on waking on three separate mornings.

Their lung function was measured with a spirometer. The primary measurement used in the analysis was the forced expiratory volume in 1 second (FEV). Vital capacity (VC) was also measured. Corrections for differences in physique were made by taking either height or VC into account.

At the end of the study it was possible not only to compare the levels of FEV between different groups of men but to determine the rate of decline in lung function over the 8 years, a statistic which cannot be obtained from a cross-sectional study. Figure 3.1 demonstrates some of the findings. The men were divided according to the number of cigarettes they smoked and, within each category, they were further grouped according to their initial level of FEV/VC (a ratio which takes into account the size of the lungs). The decline in FEV over the 8 years was very small in non-smokers and ex-smokers regardless of the initial FEV/VC value. But, with increasing smoking, increasingly steep falls in FEV were found with decreasing initial FEV/VC.

Figure 3.2 summarises these findings over the age range 25–75. Non-smokers and smokers not susceptible to smoke have a small and unimportant drop in lung function over time. Susceptible smokers have a relatively rapid fall in FEV so that they become dis-

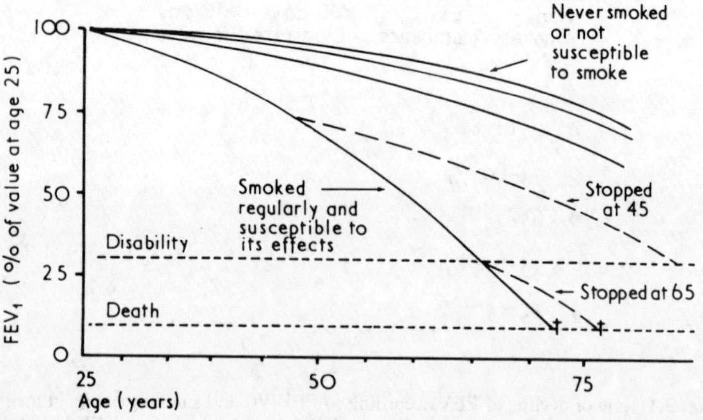

Fig. 3.2 Summary curves of decline in FEV with age for men, according to smoking habits. (From: Fletcher C M, Peto R 1977 British Medical Journal 1: 1645–8. Reproduced with the permission of the authors and the Editor of the British Medical Journal.)

abled and die prematurely. Analysis of smokers who quit indicated that, after quitting, the decline in FEV parallels the decline in non-smokers but there is no improvement in FEV level.

These longitudinal findings suggest a different interpretation to those observed in a cross-sectional study. In the latter, the effect of smoking on level of FEV may appear to be relatively small because in the non-susceptible majority of smokers it is slight and can conceal the more drastic effects on the minority of susceptible smokers. The effect may be further obscured because of misclassification of the smoking habits of heavy smokers with symptoms who tend to reduce their consumption, thus making the most susceptible smokers appear to consume relatively little tobacco.

The findings also indicated a different natural history from either the British or the Dutch hypothesis. No consistent association was found between the decline in FEV and either mucus hypersecretion or bronchial infections in both men as a group and as individuals, suggesting that neither played a part in causing irreversible airflow obstruction. The authors saw smoking as the cause of two separate conditions, chronic hypersecretion and chronic airflow obstruction.

Attributable risk. Cohort studies provide the information to calculate incidence rates. If these are calculated for those exposed and unexposed to risk factors, such as cigarette smoking, it is possible to estimate the amount of extra morbidity or mortality that may be attributed to the risk factor. This extra risk is called the attributable risk. It is commonly calculated either for the people exposed to the factor ('attributable risk of exposed persons') or for the whole population of exposed and unexposed people ('population attributable risk'). For the former, the attributable risk is the difference between the incidence rates for the exposed and unexposed groups (i.e. the 'extra' risk that the exposed have over and above the risk for the unexposed group) expressed as a proportion of the incidence rate of the exposed group. This may be written:

$$\frac{a - b}{a}$$

where a is the incidence rate for the exposed and b is the rate for the unexposed. The difference between this and the population attributable risk is that the latter takes into account the whole population, not just those exposed to the factor. Thus, even if the attributable risk is very high for exposed people, when there are very few of them in the population, the extra risk for the whole population from the exposure may be very small indeed. We return to this point again with an example in the next section.

3. Case-control studies

The advantage of the cohort over the cross-sectional study lies in its potential for defining the order in which changes occur, for determining risk factors and for estimating incidence. However the study of slowly developing chronic conditions may take many years before an answer is obtained and if the condition studied has a low incidence rate, a very large initial population may be required for enough cases to develop over a reasonable period of time. Both of these factors tend to make such studies considerably more expensive than the other designs.

The case-control design helps to overcome both these disadvantages by obtaining information about the past from people who already have the disease and comparing these patients' experiences with those of people who do not have the disease. This design is commonly used in clinical studies for which patients are usually easily accessible.

Smoking and carcinoma of the lung. In one of the classic studies in which the method was used, the relation between cigarette smoking and carcinoma of the lung was investigated (Doll & Hill, 1950). The causes of the rapid rise in lung cancer mortality in many countries during this century were not so well investigated before 1950 as they have been since that time. The main postulated causes were atmospheric pollution and tobacco smoking. The possibility of changing diagnostic habits or skills over the first half of the twentieth century was discounted as an important factor in the epidemic because the rise in mortality was found in rural as well as urban populations and in national as well as teaching hospital figures.

The study was set up to test the hypothesis that tobacco smoking was related to carcinoma of the lung. Twenty London hospitals were asked to record all patients admitted with carcinoma of the lung, stomach, colon and rectum. For each cancer patient a non-cancer control was obtained by the same hospital at or about the same time. The diagnosis at admission was later checked against diagnosis on discharge or after necropsy, if available.

Smoking histories were obtained. Anyone who admitted to smoking as much as 1 cigarette a day for as long as 1 year was classified as a smoker. The daily amount smoked immediately before the onset of disease was also recorded. It was possible then to compare the past smoking habits of lung cancer patients with those of other cancer patients and non-cancer controls. A further control group was formed by those patients originally reported to have cancer but whose diagnosis was subsequently changed. This group had the special advantage that if unrecognised biases were acting in the

Table 3.2 Number of patients with and without carcinoma of the lung according to daily average cigarettes smoked (From: Doll & Hill, 1950.)

Group	Non-smokers	Cigarette smoking: daily average					Total
		<5	5–	15–	25–	50+	
Ca lung	2	33	250	196	136	32	649
Other diseases	27	55	293	190	71	13	649
Relative risk	1.0	8.1	11.5	13.9	25.9	33.2	

selection of cancer patients who smoked, that bias should have also applied to this particular control group. Any differences in past smoking history between true cancer cases and this control group would be independent of the selection biases for cancer patients.

Table 3.2 shows some of the results for men. The distribution of smoking habits for men who had carcinoma of the lung tends to be shifted towards higher values of daily average cigarette used compared with the distribution for other patients. This might be tested using a statistic such as chi square and the difference would be found to be highly statistically significant. This would tell us that the observed differences in the way cigarette consumption was distributed between the two groups of patients would be highly unlikely to have occurred by chance. A little consideration of the numbers would lead us to say that the lung cancer patients tended to smoke more than other patients. Although this is very interesting it does not give us any idea of the difference in risk of ending up with lung cancer between smokers and non-smokers, which is what lies behind the aetiological hypothesis.

Relative risk. One of the drawbacks of the case-control study is that it cannot provide an estimate of the absolute risk of acquiring a disease or condition, since the population at risk is unknown. This may be demonstrated by considering a 2 × 2 table in which the counts of people with and without a disease are divided according to two levels of a factor. We can use the numbers from the first two columns of Table 3.2 and rearrange them into a more conventional form as in Table 3.3.

Thirty-five lung cancer patients were selected and then questioned about their past experience of cigarette smoking and 82 other patients were also selected and questioned. The absolute risk of getting cancer of the lung among the 88 smokers cannot be estimated by the ratio 33/88 because the sampling was based on the presence or absence of lung cancer, not on smoking habits. The value of the above ratio depends on the relative numbers of cases to

Table 3.3 Rearrangement of some of the data in Table 3.2 (see text)

		Cancer of the lung		
		Yes	No	Total
Smoker	Yes	33	55	88
	No	2	27	29
Total		35	82	117

controls—this is determined by the investigator and, obviously, has nothing to do with the aetiology of the disease.

But the risk of getting lung cancer in smokers relative to the risk in non-smokers can be calculated. This is known as the relative risk. The lung cancer and the non-lung cancer samples of patients are assumed to be representative of people in each of these groups and to come from the same overall population. This is an over-optimistic assumption for many reported studies, but it is no greater a methodological expectation than for cross-sectional or cohort designs. The difference in sampling between the two groups lies in the rate at which patients are selected from their populations. These rates are unknown but we could call them 1 in a for the lung cancer patients and 1 in b for the other patients—we might select 1 in 100 lung cancer patients (where $a = 100$) and 1 in 100 000 other patients (where $b = 100\,000$). The numbers we would have obtained in Table 3.3 had all patients been seen can be obtained by multiplying the number of lung cancer patients by a and the number of other patients by b. In this way we remove the effect of different sampling rates on the estimate of risk we looked at above. It can then be shown that an approximate value for the relative risk for diseases which are not very common (occurring, say, in less than 1 per cent of the population) is obtained from the ratio of the cross-products of the frequencies in the table. For Table 3.3 this value is:

$$\frac{33 \times 27}{2 \times 55} = 8.1$$

In this case smokers of less than five cigarettes a day have been found to have a risk of having lung cancer 8.1 times that of non-smokers. If there were no excess risk the value would be 1.0. Confidence limits can be calculated for the estimated relative risk to find whether they include the value 1.0. The method is not described here but the interested reader will find it in most books on medical statistics. The relative risks for each level of smoking compared with not smoking are given in Table 3.2.

Attributable risk may also be calculated for case-control studies. If r is the relative risk, then the attributable risk for exposed persons can be calculated from a formula derived from that given earlier (p. 37):

$$\frac{r - 1}{r}$$

If p is the proportion of the people in a population exposed to the risk, the population attributable risk is:

$$\frac{p\,(r - 1)}{pr + (1 - p)}$$

These may be converted to percentages by multiplying by 100.

An example will show how these risks differ in practice. Let the relative risk of lung cancer for smokers versus non-smokers be 10. The percentage of cancers in smokers attributable to smoking (the attributable risk for exposed persons) would be 100(9/10) or 90 per cent. This statistic, like the relative risk from which it is derived, is useful to the clinician as it gives an idea of the size of the effect of the risk factor on those exposed to it and the amount by which the disease might be reduced if the exposure were removed. On the other hand, the community physician is more likely to use the population attributable risk which gives an estimate of the change in the proportion of ill people in the community as a whole if the exposure were removed, say, by the use of health education or legislation. In the example if only 10 per cent of the population smoked, then the percentage of lung cancer cases in the whole population due to smoking would be 100 (0.9/(1 + 0.9)) or 47.4 per cent. If smoking were banned in this population, a reduction in lung cancer incidence by about a half might be expected.

ERROR

Error in measurement may be broadly divided into that due to random effects and that due to bias. Random error has no systematic effect on the estimation of the mean value of a set of observations because the degree to which some of the observations are above the true value is balanced by the the degree to which other observations are below the true value. On the other hand, it does increase estimations of the variability of the measurement.

In contrast, bias refers to a systematic effect on the observations. If it is constant, such as a consistent under-reading of blood pressure by 10 mmHg, then it will affect the estimate of the mean value, though not the estimate of variance. If it is not constant, it can affect both estimates, Sometimes corrections can be made to data if the amount of bias is known. Adjustments of this sort are routinely applied to laboratory tests in which the value obtained from a blank determination is subtracted from the sample value. In epidemiological studies the bias may not be measurable even if its existence is suspected. Steps must be taken to avoid it at the time of data collection.

Bias

Of the three designs so far described, that of the case-control study would seem to be the best choice for testing aetiological hypotheses since it is cheap relative to the cohort study, takes a short time for data collection and can be carried out with readily available populations such as hospital patients. Its popularity as a method for clinical investigations would support this, but the advantages are countered by notable disadvantages. There are simple ones such as the lack of standardised collection of data on past exposure to risk factors and more complicated ones which introduce biases easily overlooked by the unwary.

Well over 50 biases have been reported (Sackett, 1979) and the most important should be kept in mind. Some of these biases are also found in cross-sectional and cohort studies, as indicated below. The main biases may be divided into those introduced by sampling and those introduced by methods of measurement.

Sampling biases

Admission rate bias. One of the fundamental sampling biases which places the value of the results of case-control studies in perspective is the admission rate bias first described by Berkson (1946). This bias arises when one is dealing with a set of data with a different sampling rate for all four groups defined by the presence or absence of disease and of the factor (the four groups, for example shown in Table 3.3). It is easy to see that if the sampling rates differ in this way, the calculated value of the relative risk would depend on the relative sizes of the sampling rates. It can be shown that by such differential sampling into the four cells from a population in which there is no relation between disease and factor a highly significant association may be found in the sample obtained. Since patients and controls are often chosen in a way that precludes knowledge of differential sampling with respect to aetiological factors, there is little to be done to prevent the bias. Nevertheless the bias may be sought in part by having several independently chosen control groups. In Doll and Hill's study more than one control group was examined and a control group in which the biases of the case group might have been expected—those misdiagnosed as lung cancer—was also available. That all control groups were similar for history of cigarette smoking and differed from the lung cancer patients strengthened the likelihood that the association was genuine. Further support came from the evidence of a dose related response indicated by the increasing relative risk with increasing daily average cigarette consumption.

The prevalence-incidence bias. The prevalence-incidence bias of Neyman (1955) affects all epidemiological studies. This refers to the effect on the analysis of people who were left out of the sample because they died before they could take part, or their illness was too short for them to be included, or evidence of exposure to the causal factor was lost or the condition, though present, was clinically silent. The loss of people because of the severity of their disease and the placing of cases in the control group because of unrecognised disease are likely to weaken the observed association. Failure to determine exposure to the factor may have either a strengthening or a weakening effect; in either case it is unmeasurable. In Doll and Hill's study great attention was devoted to obtaining the smoking history. Again the increasing relative risk with dose gives some support for the belief that the retrospective exposure data were reasonably correct.

The non-response bias. The non-response bias arises because people who refuse or fail to take part in a study may be different in their characteristics from those who do take part. One well known example comes from a study of lung disease in Welsh miners. Respondents seen early in the survey tended more frequently to have evidence of pneumoconiosis, an industrial disease for which there is compensation, whereas the last group of respondents, who replied only on exhortation, tended to have tuberculosis, a disease which led to loss of occupation. The bias may be assessed by selecting a random sample of non-responders (to reduce the number to be sought out) and making a great effort to obtain their cooperation. Results from their examinations should be representative of all non-responders. In practice this is extremely difficult to do successfully. A more indirect method is to compare whatever characteristics are known of the non-responders with those of the responders and to assess the relevance of any differences to the results.

Membership bias. The membership bias refers to the self-selection of exposure by members of the case or control groups. For example, it is possible that people who have lung cancer just happen to smoke more cigarettes during their lives than those who do not have lung cancer, for reasons unrelated to cause and effect.

The unmasking bias. Finally among the sampling biases is the unmasking bias, in which new cases of the disease are unmasked by the factor under investigation but are not caused by that factor. This bias has been described for studies of the association between endometrial cancer and oestrogen therapy. Oestrogen therapy may cause uterine bleeding which then undergoes clinical investigation. Some of these women will have endometrial cancer unrelated to oestrogen therapy which has been unmasked because both disease and factor give rise to the same symptom. Thus in the analysis table analogous to that in Table 3.3, the population from which the sample in the disease-yes, factor-yes cell is drawn consists of known cases plus cases unmasked by oestrogen therapy whereas the population from which the sample in the disease-yes, factor-no cell is drawn consists only of known cases. This violates the assumption made earlier that the cases were drawn at random from all cases and may lead to serious errors in estimating relative risk. This bias may be prevented by matching cases and controls on method of detection.

Measurement biases

Recall bias and family information bias. Measurement biases may be introduced by respondents. Recall bias may exaggerate the differences in exposure between cases and controls because having the case condition may sharpen the memory for events or exposures which might be causative. Family information bias also arises from selective memory or experience. Cases may remember the occurrence of their own disease in other family members or may have been told of the disease in the family because they themselves had it whereas siblings or close relatives without the disease may have forgotten or never known of the family history. This bias is of profound importance in family studies. Its existence can be detected by gathering factual information about the family from medical records, registers or other records independent of the case's memory.

Exposure suspicion bias. Exposure suspicion bias is introduced by the observer. If the interviewer, fieldworker or whoever is collecting the data suspects that the respondent has been exposed to the factor of interest, he may investigate the respondent to a greater extent than if no such suspicion existed. This bias may be reduced or eliminated by carefully structuring the way in which the data are collected and by training fieldworkers to make the collection in a systematic way.

The diagnostic suspicion bias. The diagnostic suspicion bias is similar to the exposure suspicion bias but does not play an important part in case-control studies. It can affect the results of cohort studies, however, because the diagnosis of a condition is made in previously healthy people. If the diagnosis is suspected, then that respondent may be more closely investigated than other respondents. Because different criteria for diagnosis are used for those under suspicion compared with those who are not, the condition in one group is not the same as in the other. This bias may be countered by using well-designed criteria for diagnosis to be applied to all respondents.

All the measurement biases tend to increase the differences between the cases and controls. In cross-sectional and cohort studies only the diagnostic suspicion bias is important; the others either have little effect or are inapplicable. However, in these study types instrument bias is of particular concern. Instruments should obviously be properly calibrated and maintained so they give accurate and reliable readings. Drift in calibration techniques or reference standards may lead to misinterpretation of time trends or the natural history of the disease and must be avoided or minimised. Observer bias will also affect readings from instruments or the results from questionnaires administered by interviewers. The measurement of blood pressure by the standard mercury sphygmomanometer is particularly subject to observer bias. Lowe & McKeown (1962), among others, have shown that if an observer overestimates systolic blood pressure, this is no indication of how he will read diastolic pressure. They also showed that observers have a preference for recording values ending in a 0 rather than 5. Preconceived ideas of the dividing line between normotension and hypertension may lead to an unconscious avoidance of recording values at the cut-off levels—presumably to avoid the clinical uncertainty they imply.

Observer bias may be reduced or even eliminated by careful training of the observers and monitoring the comparability of the measurements and the use of instruments such as the random zero sphygmomanometer which are designed to limit the influence of the observer.

Even in the best planned study there will be biases, some of them unknown and unavoidable. Acceptance of the results of a single study should therefore be guarded unless the evidence is overwhelming. If a large number of studies using different designs and methods all come to the same conclusion, the likelihood that a true association has been found is much increased. But even this may be insufficient, as positive results tend to be more readily published than negative ones.

To help in reaching a conclusion, Bradford Hill (1965) suggested criteria for determining whether a causal interpretation is likely. The association should be judged on its:

1. Strength, which may be measured by the relative risk, correlation coefficient or other appropriate statistic.
2. Consistency, that is it should be observed in several studies using different populations and methods.
3. Specificity to a particular population group (one sex, a limited age range, one ethnic group etc.) and type of disease.
4. Temporality; the suspected cause should be observed to act on the population before a change in health occurs.
5. Dose-response curve.
6. Biological plausibility; it should have an explanation based on current biological knowledge.
7. Coherence; it should not conflict with other known facts about the natural history of the disease.
8. Support from experimental evidence.
9. Support from analogous biological associations.

Some of these criteria obviously carry more weight than others and the more that are fulfilled by the results of an investigation, the stronger is the case for causality. Nevertheless, even when all are met, causality is not proven but only strongly supported.

SAMPLING

Having defined the question to be asked, chosen a population to study and selected a study design, the researcher must decide how to take a sample from the population. In epidemiological studies, units of a population are often people, but a 'population' can consist of all sorts of units such as metropolitan boroughs, the present day equivalent of the county boroughs (used in studies of the geographical distribution of mortality), hospitals or any other entity in some defined grouping. In some cases the population may be sufficiently small that every member can be studied. If this is impractical because the population is too large, then a sample of its members must be drawn. Results from the sample should represent the situation in the whole population.

If the investigator chooses his sample at his own discretion it is unlikely to be representative of the whole population. He may, for convenience, choose volunteers or those who happen to be in a particular place at a particular time. 'Grab' sampling in this way means that the population from which the sample is taken is unknown so its representativeness cannot be judged. The biases can be avoided by using methods which remove from the investigator the decision of who enters the study.

A sampling frame is required. This is a list of the members of the population from which the sample is to be drawn. Various ready-made frames are available such as the electoral roll or a general practitioner's list of patients. Several methods are used for sampling from the frame.

Random sampling is used to obtain an unbiased sample representative of the whole population. To choose at random means that every individual has an equal chance of entering the sample. In the simple random sample every member in the frame is given a unique number from one to the number of members. Using a table of random numbers (created by selecting digits at random and found as published tables or obtained by computer) a sample of numbers is drawn and matched with the numbers on the list. These selected individuals form the sample.

The stratified random sample is one in which simple random samples are drawn from within defined groups (strata) of the sampling frame. The sampling rates will differ between groups so that the number of selected people in small groups will be sufficient for useful analysis. The method also allows a more precise estimate of the values in the whole population by ensuring that people in the small groups are represented in whatever sample is drawn. The cohort study of chronic bronchitis described above used stratified sampling so that there would be enough men in the sample of those with symptoms. The authors chose all those who had admitted to having chest symptoms in a screening questionnaire, half of those who were asymptomatic non-smokers and a fifth of those who were asymptomatic smokers and ex-smokers. All the symptomatic men were chosen as this was the group in which the greatest change in FEV was expected and would thus provide most information on the natural history of a chronic condition over a short time. A relatively high proportion of asymptomatic non-smokers was taken because there were not very many of them (only 282 out of 3013 men).

Systematic sampling, which is much less laborious than random sampling, is often used when the sampling frame is already listed, such as the patients signed up with a general practitioner. The size of both the list and the desired sample must be known so that the sampling fraction can be calculated (sample size/list size). If, for example, the list size is 1000 people from whom 100 are needed for the sample, the sampling fraction would be 1 in 10. One person in the first 10 on the list should be chosen at random and then every 10th person further down the list is taken into the sample until the list is exhausted. If there are cyclical changes in step with the sampling fraction (e.g. every 10th person might be female because of the way the records are kept) the sample may have characteristics which differ greatly from those of the population from which it was drawn. But, provided such changes are avoided, the sample should not be biased.

Other methods of sampling are used depending on the circumstances and the sort of frame available. Cluster sampling is useful when the individuals can only be enumerated as a group such as a village or a place of work. Analysis of cluster samples may be more complex than for either the simple or stratified samples particularly since the standard package computer programs are not written for this method of sampling.

ASSESSING THE QUALITY OF MEASUREMENT

Measurements used in community studies, whatever they are, need to be as accurate and repeatable as possible. Many techniques have been assessed before they are used by the epidemiologist so it is unnecessary to repeat the assessment each time they are used in a new study, but new measuring instruments, particularly questionnaires, may be needed and these must be tested to determine how good they are.

The instrument or test must be valid, that is, it must measure the thing it is expected to measure. The test used in the survey may be a simplified form of a test too time consuming or complex to apply to large numbers of people. The results of the simple test are compared with the results of the complex test which may be thought of as giving the true answer (though it too may be found to be in error when a more accurate test is developed). Two groups of people are used to test the simple test, one made up of those positive to the true, complex test and the other of those who are negative. Each group is then tested with the simple test. If the simple test is completely valid then it will be positive in all those who have a positive complex test and it will be negative in those with a negative complex test. This does not occur in practice; there will always be some false negatives and some false positives. The statistics used for measuring validity, specificity and sensitivity, show to what extent the simple test gives false results.

Table 3.4 shows the calculation of these two values using data

Table 3.4 Reported hearing difficulty in men related to deafness defined by results of an audiogram. (D'Souza et al 1975 Journal of the Royal College of General Practitioners 25: 472–478.)

Test		Audiogram result Deaf	Not deaf
Reported hearing difficulty	Yes	33	98
	No	19	935
Total		52	1033

Specificity = 935/1033 = 90.5%.
Sensitivity = 33/52 = 63.5%

from a study of screening for deafness. Patients in a general practice were given a questionnaire to complete which asked a set of standard questions about their hearing. The validity of the questions on hearing difficulty was assessed by comparing the answers with audiogram results. The audiogram was thought of as providing a true result against which the more simple test of a questionnaire was evaluated. Specificity in this example is the percentage of not deaf people who answered no to the questions (935/1033 or 91 per cent.) This means that 5 per cent of not deaf people falsely reported themselves to have hearing difficulties. The table shows that the questionnaire when used in this particular population picked out three times as many false positives as true positives (deaf people who answered yes to the questionnaire)! Sensitivity is the percentage of deaf people who answered yes to the questions (33/52 or 63.5 per cent). In this study the sensitivity was rather low, implying that many of the audiometrically deaf were not identified by the questionnaire.

Real-life values for sensitivity of good tests are likely to lie between 80 and 100 per cent. For epidemiological purposes, when most people surveyed are likely to be negative, the specificity should be of the order of 97 per cent or more because, if less, there may be far more false positives than true positives to the simple test. In the example, the questionnaire turned out to be an unsatisfactory way of identifying the deaf. Both its sensitivity and specificity were too low to be useful.

Reliability of the measurement must also be assessed. Reliability refers to the ability of the measuring device to give the same results when used more than once and by more than one observer. There are a number of ways of calculating a value for reliability. One way is illustrated in Table 3.5. This shows the agreement between two radiologists on whether or not to refer a patient after assessing her

Table 3.5 Agreement between two radiologists interpreting mammograms on the need to refer women for a surgical opinion. (From: Chamberlain J et al 1975 Lancet ii: 1026–30)

Radiologist A	Radiologist B	
	Referral	No referral
Referral	39	13
No referral	24	1138

Agreement on referrals = 39/(39 + 13 + 24) = 51%.

mammogram in a study of screening for breast cancer. The agreement was calculated as the number of women who would have been referred by both radiologists as a percentage of the total number of referrals (39/76 or 51 per cent). Other statistics may also be used and the reader is referred to more specialised books for these.

The reader is referred for a more detailed and highly readable discussion of diagnostic tests to two articles from the Department of Clinical Epidemiology and Biostatistics at McMaster University (1980; 1981).

CONCLUSION

In this chapter we have tried to show how problems are tackled in population research. The idea for a research project may come from almost any source but it is up to the researcher to formulate the researchable questions. This process may be helped by considering the problem in terms of an equation in which the outcome variable is predicted by a set of other variables.

Once the hypothesis has been defined, and this may take some time and argument, the study design can be chosen which best fits the problem and the practical constraints such as available populations and financial resources. The methods of measurement must be selected and new ones must be assessed for validity and repeatability. Observers must be trained to use the instruments and the questionnaire to avoid introducing their own personal biases.

A suitable population should be selected for which there is a sampling frame, whether ready-made or created by private census. The sampling method must be chosen and the method of analysis outlined.

The process of measuring a problem is not a straight forward step-by-step procedure. Decisions made early in the process may need revision in the light of later thoughts. The preparation of the plans of a study should be by a multidisciplinary team including an experienced statistician. The statistician will help with determining the required sample size, the method of sampling, data preparation methods and analysis.

REFERENCES

Berkson J 1946 Limitations of the application of fourfold table analysis to hospital data. Biometrics Bulletin 2: 47–53

Chinn S, Florey C duV, Baldwin I G, Gorgol M 1981 The relation of mortality in England and Wales 1969–73 to measurements of air pollution. Journal of Epidemiology and Community Health 35: 174–179

Daly C 1959 Air pollution and causes of death. British Journal of Preventive and Social Medicine 13: 14–27

Department of Clinical Epidemiology and Biostatistics, McMaster University, Hamilton, Ont. 1980 Clinical disagreement: I. How often it occurs and why. Canadian Medical Association Journal 123: 499–504

Department of Clinical Epidemiology and Biostatistics, McMaster University Health Sciences Centre 1981 How to read clinical journals: II. To learn about a diagnostic test. Canadian Medical Association Journal 124: 703–10

Doll R, Hill A B 1950 Smoking and carcinoma of the lung. British Medical Journal ii: 739–48

Ferris B G, Higgins I T T, Higgins M W, Peters J M 1973 Chronic nonspecific respiratory disease in Berlin, New Hampshire, 1961 to 1967. A follow-up study. American Review of Respiratory Diseases 107: 110–22

Fletcher C, Peto R, Tinker C, Speizer F E 1976 The natural history of chronic bronchitis and emphysema. Oxford University Press, Oxford

Gardner M J, Crawford M D, Morris J N 1969 Patterns of morbidity in middle and early old age in the county boroughs of England and Wales. British Journal of Preventive and Social Medicine 23: 133–40

Hill A B 1965 The environment and disease: association or causation? Proceedings of the Royal Society of Medicine 58: 295–300

Lowe C R, McKeown T 1962 Arterial pressure in an industrial population and its bearing on the problem of essential hypertension. Lancet i: 1086–92

Lunn J E, Knowelden J, Handyside A J 1967 Patterns of respiratory illness in Sheffield infant schoolchildren. British Journal of Preventive and Social Medicine 21: 7–16

Neyman J 1955 Statistics—servant of all sciences. Science 122: 401

Sackett D 1979 Bias in analytic research. Journal of Chronic Diseases 32: 51–63

FURTHER READING

Alderson M 1976 An introduction to epidemiology. MacMillan, London
This book describes in considerable detail with many examples the uses of routinely collected data and the design of epidemiological studies.

Barker DJP, Rose G 1979 Epidemiology in medical practice, 2nd edn. Churchill Livingstone, Edinburgh
A short book covering many of the points made in Chapter 3 but in greater detail. It also discusses description of disease in the community and some aspects of the application of epidemiological methods to patient care.

Friedman GD 1974 Primer of epidemiology. McGraw-Hill, New York
Basic descriptions of epidemiological studies and practical advice on how to do a study are given.

4

Treatment and prevention: the options for action

INTRODUCTION: EFFICACY AND EFFECTIVENESS

Community medicine is concerned not only with describing problems and disentangling causes, but also with providing and evaluating solutions to those problems. The solutions of community medicine are, however, different from the solutions of clinical, or bedside, medicine. In clinical medicine the prime concern is with the individual patient who attends for help. This puts the responsibility on the doctor to ensure that the procedure that he prescribes has been shown to be 'efficacious' in properly controlled trials. Efficacy in this sense means that the procedure or drug does what it is designed to do when applied to an individual patient. For instance, in prescribing for a hypertensive patient the doctor will want to know that the drug prescribed is likely to lower the blood pressure without unwanted side-effects, and that this treatment will favourably affect the prognosis of the patient.

The central question in community medicine is not whether a procedure administered to a suitable patient will have a beneficial effect on that patient, but whether the service that is provided for a community is having a beneficial effect on that community. If a service does this it is described as 'effective'. An effective service depends on the application of efficacious procedures, but this is not enough. To ensure that the service is effective the procedures must reach those who would benefit from them and be safe.

Medical progress is often portrayed in terms of new and more efficacious treatments but such a view is inadequate. A large proportion of medical problems can already be prevented or treated. The difficulty is in ensuring that such treatments are effective at a community level. The elimination of smallpox was achieved more than two centuries after the discovery of a relatively safe and efficacious vaccine because it was not until the 1970s that the ability to organise a worldwide preventive strategy was achieved. Trachoma is caused by an organism that is susceptible to several antibiotics.

Yet, though sulphonamides have been in use since the 1930s, 500 000 000 people suffer from this disease worldwide and 2 000 000 are blind from it. To take an example closer to home, over 80 per cent of lung cancer in the UK is due to smoking tobacco, mostly as cigarettes, yet tobacco sales remain high and in 1978 34 000 people died of this disease in England and Wales alone.

CURATIVE SERVICES

Effectiveness

In order to be effective a health care programme must use safe and efficacious procedures, and it must distribute care to those who need it. Both of these requirements are of importance to community medicine.

Efficacy and safety

The first requirement for an effective service is that the procedures used are both efficacious and safe. As this cannot always be assumed, efficacy and safety inevitably become subjects of importance in community medicine. In 1969 the Sainsbury Committee of Enquiry into the Relationship of the Pharmaceutical Industry with the National Health Service classified the 2657 preparations listed in the Monthly Index of Medical Specialties (MIMS) as follows:

50 per cent	Therapeutically effective preparations
35 per cent	Undesirable preparations
8 per cent	Rational combinations
7 per cent	Not yet classified

That such a small proportion of pharmaceuticals was found to be efficacious was worrying, but the dangers from side-effects are even more serious than the prescription of spurious cures. Accidental poisoning by drugs and medicaments accounted for 528 deaths in England and Wales in 1978. A further 85 deaths were certified as being due to surgical and medical complications and misadventures. This takes no account of the non-fatal morbidity ascribed to the prescription of drugs. Davies (1977) has estimated that 10–20 per cent of those prescribed drugs suffer some side-effect, and that 3–5 per cent of those admitted to hospital are admitted primarily because of an adverse reaction to a drug. In a number of studies the mortality from adverse drug reactions has been estimated as anything up to 3 per 1000 inpatients.

The distribution of care

Availability of care. Given the existence of an efficacious treatment, the single most important barrier to receiving it is the overall supply or availability. This is most marked where a new treatment is first introduced. Figure 4.1 shows the number of patients being treated for chronic renal failure between 1971 and 1980. As the dialysis service and transplant programme developed, so the numbers being treated increased.

Even where a treatment is well established, however, there are often financial constraints on how much of the technology is provided, and these depend on how much the country is able or willing to spend on health care in general, and on any specified programme in particular. This subject will be dealt with in greater detail in Chapter 6.

Access to care. Even where a service is available, the use that is made of it is not always in direct proportion to the apparent need for it. This has led to the conclusion that there are barriers to access. The barriers that have been suggested are physical such as distance from a treatment centre or poor transport facilities, economic where there is a fee charged or where wages are lost when attending the service, and cultural. It is not always easy to tell which of these theoretical barriers is operating in any particular situation.

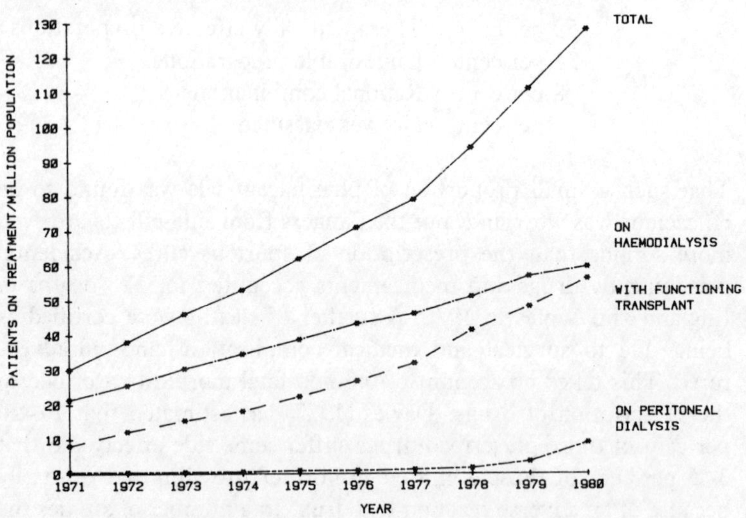

Fig. 4.1 Treatment for chronic renal failure in the UK, 1971–80 (Based on information from the European Dialysis and Transplant Association.)

Inequality of use

Social class. The inequality in the uptake of services that has created most controversy is that between social classes. The introduction of the National Health Service was seen as a way of reducing the disparity between need for and access to services by ensuring that everyone could obtain treatment without payment at the time that they needed it. Financial barriers are not the only reason for lower uptake among poor people; differences in knowledge and perceptions are also important, particularly in the uptake of preventive services.

In Britain now there seems to be little consistent trend in the uptake of primary health care from one social class to another. Figure 4.2 shows data collected by the General Household Survey in 1974. After standardising for age structure and the amount of sickness experienced, manual social classes do not make less use of their general practitioners than non-manual social classes. There is a tendency for unskilled manual workers (social class V) to use primary health services less, but this deficit is almost entirely due to a lower uptake by those who have a chronic sickness with consequent restriction of activities. For chronic sickness without restriction of activity and for acute sickness there is a consistent increase in service uptake from social class II to social class V.

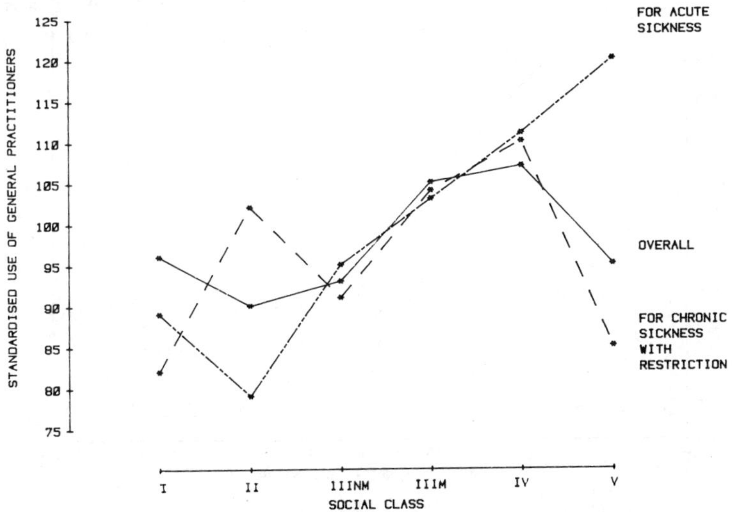

Fig. 4.2 Uptake of GP services by social class and type of sickness. (Based on: Collins E, Klein R 1980 Equity and NHS: self reported morbidity, access and primary care. British Medical Journal 281: 1111–5)

Old age. The same data show that those above 65 years of age consult the doctor less than those who are younger, given the same type of sickness. Although this may imply that less care is given to the elderly, it is more likely that the elderly need to go to the doctor less often for purely administrative reasons. A man of working age has to go to the doctor to get a sickness certificate regardless of whether he thinks the doctor can do anything to cure him. After retirement this is no longer necessary.

Distance. Even within the narrow confines of a London general practice it is possible to observe differences in consultation rates between those living close to the practice, and those living further away (Parkin, 1979). The proportion of home visits also decreases with distance from the practice, and this difference in consultation rates is more marked among the elderly. Men of working age and members of social classes I and II, on the other hand, show no tendency to consult less if they live further from the practice.

This effect is comparatively small in London but is very marked elsewhere. Figure 4.3 shows the distribution of registered patients on anti-tuberculous chemotherapy in a rural area surrounding a district hospital in Africa. The number of patients falls off exponentially as distance from the hospital increases, whereas the number

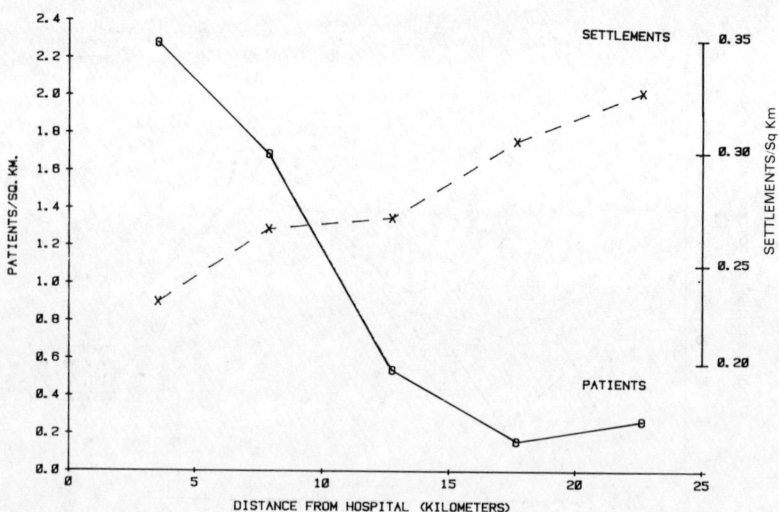

Fig. 4.3 Care gradient for tuberculosis outpatients attending St Lucy's Hospital, Transkei. (From: Burney P G J, Shahyar S 1980 Tuberculosis in the Transkei. In: Wilson F, Westcott G (eds) Economics of health in South Africa. II: Hunger, work and health. Ravan Press, Johannesburg.)

of settlements increases. The effectiveness of the treatment of tuberculosis will also be inversely related to distance from the hospital.

The inverse care law and the quality of medical care
Although consultation rates are broadly similar for different social classes, there is evidence that inequalities do persist in the distribution of health service resources. In 1971 Hart formulated his 'Inverse care law':

> In areas with most sickness and death, general practitioners have more work, larger lists, less hospital support, and inherit more clinically ineffective traditions of consultation, than in the healthiest areas; and hospital doctors shoulder heavier case-loads with less staff and equipment, more obsolete buildings, and suffer recurrent crises in the availability of beds and in the replacement of staff. These trends can be summed up as the inverse care law: that the availability of good medical care tends to vary inversely with the need of the population served. (Hart, 1971).

Information on expenditure in the National Health Service confirms this picture. Figure 4.4 shows the expenditure on community health services in regions according to what proportion of the population is in social classes IV and V. There is an obvious

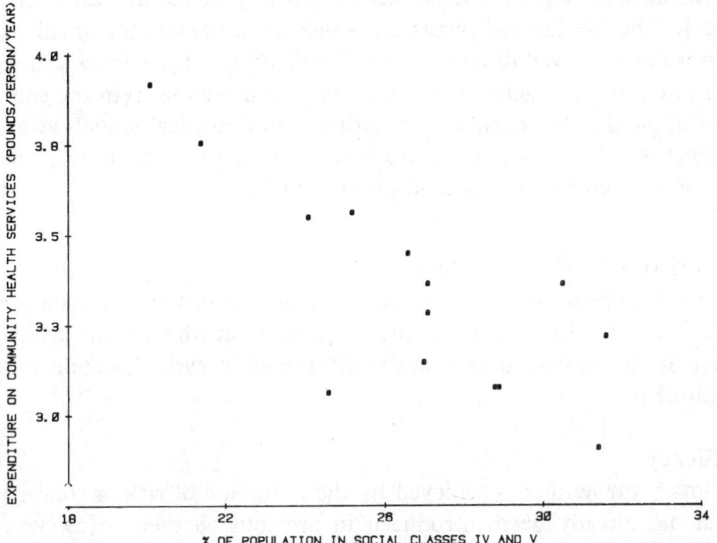

Fig. 4.4 Expenditure on community health services in 14 regions according to proportion of population in social classes IV and V. (Based on information from: Noyce J, Trickey A J, Snaith A H 1974 Regional variations in the allocation of resources to the community health services. Lancet 1: 554–7.)

trend for those regions with a higher proportion of manual social class residents to have lower expenditure on community health services.

The effect of this on the health of the population is hard to evaluate. There is evidence that teaching hospitals have lower case fatality rates than district general hospitals for a number of conditions. On the other hand more detailed studies on the prognosis for hyperplasia of the prostate have shown among other things that the teaching hospitals have patients with an initially better prognosis. Their admission is more often routine rather than as an emergency, they are younger, and have more favourable medical and social circumstances (Ashley et al, 1971).

The maldistribution of resources is a common problem in health systems throughout the world. The main corrective is in planning the distribution of services to take account of need. This is done not only in the overall budgeting, but also in giving financial incentives to doctors to work in less favoured areas and sometimes also in restricting their right to practise in 'overdoctored' areas. In the UK general practice has been regulated in this way, though probably to little effect (Butler & Knight, 1975). In 'designated' underdoctored areas GPs are given a financial incentive to practise, while special permission is required before setting up in practice in 'restricted' areas. The 'designated' areas allowance is, however, too small to offset the perceived disadvantages of practising in these areas which are often in unattractive neighbourhoods and remote from the centres of medical 'excellence'. The siting of new medical schools away from the older medical centres has been adopted as one way of trying to overcome this second disadvantage.

PRIMARY PREVENTION

Primary prevention is the avoidance of disease in the first instance and is distinguished from secondary prevention which is the avoidance of the consequences of advanced disease by early detection and treatment.

Efficacy

Primary prevention is achieved by the reduction of risk, a concept that has already been introduced in previous chapters. However, not every risk factor is causally related to the disease with which it is associated and if there is no causal relation, no amount of 'risk reduction' will result in the prevention of disease. Table 4.1 gives some of the results of a randomised controlled trial of giving advice not to smoke in pregnancy. It is well established that the children of women who smoke have a lower birth weight than the children of women who do not smoke. But the results of the trial failed to show any advantage to those women who were given the intensive health education during pregnancy though the advice appears to have resulted in a lower prevalence of smoking among the mothers given the advice. If we assume that the mothers in the treatment group really did give up smoking, there are at least two possible explanations for this. First, advice not to smoke given in early pregnancy may come too late, either because the effect of smoking occurs early in pregnancy, or because the effect lasts beyond the time at which the woman gives up smoking. Alternatively, although the women in each group entering this trial appeared very similar in terms of initial smoking habits, age, date of booking, height, parity, social class and education, it may be that smoking is not the factor that directly affects the birth weight of the baby, but some other confounding factor that has not been measured and which is associated with smoking. In either case, though the health education programme is tackling a risk factor that is known to be associated with low birth weight, namely smoking during pregnancy, it is not tackling the factor that causes low birth weight, namely smoking in the months before pregnancy, smoking in early pregnancy, or an unknown factor associated with smoking.

Table 4.1 Some results from a randomised trial of anti-smoking advice in pregnancy (Standard errors are given in parentheses). (From: Donovan JW 1977 Randomised controlled trial of anti-smoking advice in pregnancy. British Journal of Preventive Medicine 31: 6–12.)

	Treatment group			
	Test (263)		Control (289)	
Cigarettes smoked per day				
Before pregnancy	19.7	(0.6)	18.3	(0.5)
Early pregnancy	17.1	(0.6)	14.7	(0.4)
Mid pregnancy	12.1	(0.5)	14.7	(0.6)
Late pregnancy	9.2	(0.6)	16.4	(0.6)
Measurements taken at maturity (days)	280.8	(1.1)	280.4	(1.0)
Weight (g)	3172	(35)	3184	(30)
% Below 2500 g	10		9	
% Born before 36 weeks	6		6	
Head circumference (cm)	34.6	(0.1)	34.7	(0.1)
Crown rump length (cm)	33.9	(0.1)	33.8	(0.2)
Crown heel length (cm)	49.7	(0.2)	49.8	(0.1)
Placental weight (g)	646	(9)	651	(8)
% Liveborn passing meconium	16		17	
Perinatal deaths	4		1	

Relative risk and population attributable risk

The effectiveness of any prophylactic service will depend on the efficacy of the procedures that it adopts. It will also depend on the distribution of its effect in the population. This distribution depends in turn on the size of the population attributable risk that is to be reduced and on whether the measures affect the general population, or whether they affect only individuals.

Table 4.2 shows the risks associated with different methods of road transport in England and Wales. Compared with car drivers a pedal cyclist travelling the same distance has 13 times the risk of sustaining a serious injury or of being killed (relative risk = 13). A doctor giving advice to a pedal cyclist on how to reduce his risk of accidental death could recommend that his patient should in future go by car. A motor-cyclist takes a risk 32 times that of the car driver, and might be advised to go by any other means of transport.

From the perspective of the community physician, however, the situation appears very different. The central issue is not reduction of the risk to an individual, but reduction of the aggregate risk to the whole population. Looked at from this perspective, the commonest cause of serious accidents is the car, followed closely by the motor-cycle; compared to these the pedal cycle is a trivial problem. Though for every mile travelled pedal cyclists are involved in 13 times as many serious accidents as car drivers, far more people travel by car. Therefore a small reduction in the already small risk to those travelling by car will result in a far greater fall in the number of injuries sustained than even the total abolition of injuries sustained in accidents to pedal cyclists. One estimate for instance suggests that an increase in seatbelt use to 85 per cent by front seat passengers in Britain would lead to a fall in fatal and serious in-

Table 4.2 Deaths and serious injuries from road traffic accidents in Great Britain, 1976. (From: Social Trends No. 8, 1977.)

Type of vehicle	Killed and seriously injured	Deaths and serious injuries/ 100 million vehicle km
Pedal cyclist	4900	126
Two-wheeled motor vehicles	17 900	308
Four-wheeled motor vehicles	22 100	
Cars and taxis		10
Goods vehicles		6
Public service vehicles		4

juries of 13 000 per annum, an effect equivalent to over two and a half times the total effect if all risk to pedal cyclists were abolished.

General intervention

There are a number of risk factors that an individual is unable to change for himself. In these cases, if any preventive measures are to be taken, they must be taken by the community as a whole and this, in general, means government action.

Outside air pollution in the 1950s was primarily due to the burning of coal on domestic fires and emissions from industrial sources. An individual convinced that this pollution was bad for his health who burnt smokeless fuel would not substantially reduce his chances of developing chronic lung disease. The Clean Air Act of 1956 enabled the designation of smokeless zones and effectively reduced air pollution by restricting the use of any fuel except smokeless fuel in those areas.

The actions of other members of the community are not the only limitation on an individual's ability to reduce risks; these are also financial constraints. Hypothermia is a common problem among the elderly. In one national survey in the UK 10 per cent of a sample of old people had a deep body temperature of less than 35.3°C (Fox et al, 1973). Although the aetiology of this condition may involve disturbances of the central mechanisms for regulatory control, a diminishing ability to sense cold, poor mobility and hypothyroidism, a constant feature for a large proportion of those affected is poverty and the problem is exacerbated by the high cost of heating fuel. The individuals concerned had no way of influencing either of these factors, but government was able to intervene by introducing a fuel allowance for the elderly.

While government restricts itself to reducing those risks that individuals cannot reduce for themselves, its actions are mostly uncontroversial. There are times, however, when it intervenes to enforce preventive measures which primarily reduce only the risks to those on whom the measures are imposed. There are two reasons given for doing this. First, where the costs of the disease are not entirely borne by the individual, it is argued that government has a right to intervene. Second, legislation ensures that those who are in greatest need are affected by the measures, and ignorance or poor access to information will not be a barrier to the benefits of prevention.

Immunisation primarily protects the individual who is immunised. However, infectious diseases, particularly those that spread from one individual to another, depend on there being sufficient susceptible individuals in the population for their spread to take place. An individual is able to protect himself by being immunised, but if a large part of a community, generally thought to be about 80 per cent, is immunised, there will be so few susceptibles in the community that the disease will not become established in the few that are left. The effect of immunisation is therefore potentially greater than the sum of the protection given to each individual: this effect is known as 'herd immunity'. Herd immunity has two important consequences. First, a disease such as smallpox can be eradicated even though not every individual in the world has been vaccinated. Second, where there are some individuals who, for whatever reason, cannot be immunised, these individuals can still be protected if all the other members of their community are immunised. For instance, children with a history of convulsions should not be given pertussis vaccine, but whooping-cough is at least as dangerous for them as for other children. The only way that they can be protected from the disease without running the unacceptable risks of immunisation is by a high uptake of vaccine among those children who can receive it safely.

No vaccine is currently compulsory in the UK, though back in 1854 Parliament, which then had a strong non-interventionist bias, passed a Vaccination Act which made smallpox vaccine compulsory for all infants. It did so largely on the advice of Sir John Simon who argued that a man indulging a preference for smallpox, did so to the detriment of his neighbour. In some countries immunisation is still compulsory, and is made a condition of entry into primary school.

As the cost of treatment is increasingly borne by central funds it is argued that the state has a right to insist on individuals taking reasonable precautions. This argument has been used, for instance, in the debate over whether wearing seatbelts should be made compulsory, even though their use has no effect on anyone but the wearer.

The second reason given for governments interfering in the risks which individuals take is that compulsion ensures that the reduction in risk is spread evenly throughout the community, especially to those at greatest risk. Deprived groups who have worse health are less likely to value or to use preventive services or to alter their behaviour in order to avoid risks. For instance in Britain, members of social class V are more likely to smoke, less likely to breast feed, less likely to have their babies immunised, less likely to take their children to the dentist, and less likely to attend child health clinics.

In the UK, government has approved the fluoridation of drink-

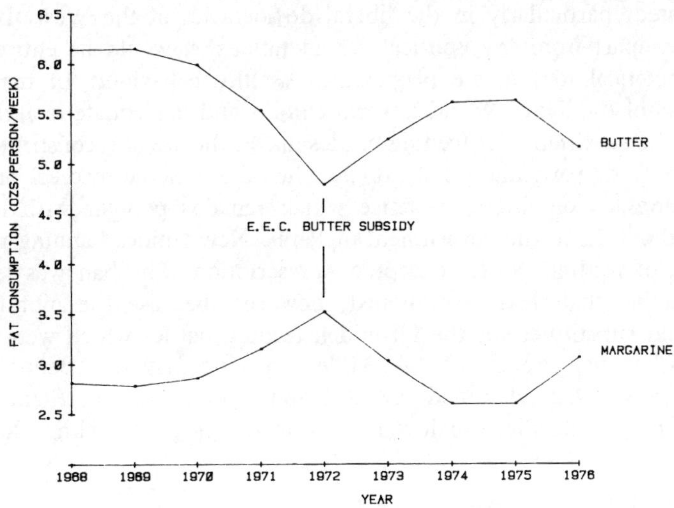

Fig. 4.5 Fat consumption in Great Britain 1968–75. (Adapted from: Florey C du V, Melia R J W, Darby S C 1978 Changing mortality from ischaemic heart disease in Great Britain. British Medical Journal 1: 635–7.)

ing water on these grounds, though it is quite possible for individuals to ensure an adequate intake of fluoride for themselves. Areas where the drinking water has a concentration of less than one part per million of fluoride experience a high incidence of dental decay. Where the deficiency has been made good by the addition of fluoride, the incidence of caries has fallen. Although central government policy is that all drinking water should have a minimum fluoride level, local opposition has in fact prevented many authorities from carrying out this policy.

Finally, government action affects health even when this is not the prime motive behind the action. The excise duty on tobacco and alcohol probably affects their consumption; though the main motive is to raise revenue this probably also affects health. In order to assist dairy farmers the EEC has subsidised butter and (Fig. 4.5) the consequent fall in butter prices relative to the price of margarine has increased the sales of butter. As it is currently believed that a diet high in saturated fats has an adverse effect on health, in this instance government may well have taken action that will damage health.

Health education: intervention at the level of the individual

Government intervention in an individual's affairs, even where that intervention is intended to be in his best interest, is generally mistrusted, particularly in the liberal democracies of the West. But even apart from any political considerations, it would be entirely impractical to regulate people into healthy behaviour. In many parts of the Third World a warm climate and inadequate facilities for the sterilisation of feeding bottles makes the use of reconstituted milk feeds particularly hazardous. The failure of the medical profession to contain the practice which remains popular with the mothers led to the government of Papua New Guinea banning the sale of feeding bottles except on prescription. The ban was less effective than had been hoped, however, because the mothers found substitutes for the forbidden feeding bottles which were at least as dangerous. To take a less specific instance, Belloc & Breslow (1972) identified seven attributes in a study in Alameda County, California, which were associated with good health. These were:

1. Eating breakfast every day
2. Not taking snacks between meals
3. Taking moderate exercise two to three times each day
4. Not smoking
5. Drinking no alcohol, or drinking alcohol in moderation
6. Not being overweight
7. Having 7–8 hours sleep each night.

Although those obeying all seven of these rules had an expectation of life 11 years longer than those who did not, it is hard to imagine what sort of regulations could be devised to enforce such exemplary behaviour, or what arrangements could be made to police them. Nor could these seven rules of healthy living be regarded as exhaustive. Nevertheless, if people cannot be regulated into a healthy lifestyle they may still be educated to choose one of their own accord.

There is no doubt that health education can be effective. Table 4.3 shows the results from a trial of health education designed to persuade men to give up smoking after surviving a myocardial infarction. The intensive health education was more effective than the usual advice that was given to all the patients. On a wider scale the Health Education Council launched a campaign in 1974 to stop women smoking in pregnancy. At the beginning of the campaign 39 per cent of pregnant women were smoking. By the end of the campaign the prevalence had declined to 29 per cent, a 26 per cent fall in the prevalence of smoking in this group of women, and an important change. But awareness of the dangers of smoking had only

Table 4.3 Some results from a trial of intensive anti-smoking advice following myocardial infarction (From: Burt A, Illingworth D, Shaw T R D, Thornley P, White P, Turner R 1974 Stopping smoking after myocardial infarction. Lancet 1: 304–6.)

Change in smoking habits	Intensive advice (125)	Conventional advice (98)
% No change	15.2	45.0
% Reduced	21.6	27.5
% Stopped	63.2	27.5
	100.0	100.0

risen from 76 to 80 per cent, a comparatively small change, highlighting one of the ambiguities of health education.

Health education may impart knowledge, but to be effective it must also change behaviour. The Health Education Council's campaign failed to change knowledge but had a modest success in altering behaviour. A similar lack of association between knowledge and behaviour has been noted in other studies. A comparison of medical students and law students in Manchester showed that although the medical students knew more about the dangers of smoking and assessed the evidence for the dangers of smoking as more convincing, it was the law students who were less likely to take up smoking (Knopf & Wakefield, 1974).

One of the advantages claimed for health education over regulation by government is that health education imparts knowledge and leaves the individual free to choose. The disparity between increasing knowledge and altering behaviour, and the priority usually given to changing behaviour in health education, threatens to undermine this advantage. In order to alter behaviour the methods used by health education may become increasingly intrusive. Hilary Graham (1976) has studied women who smoke in pregnancy. Some women have heard that smoking is bad during pregnancy, and yet continue to smoke. Some of these mothers dismiss the 'scientific' evidence out of hand. They see 'science' as being irrelevant, providing information that is not confirmed by everyday experience in their own lives or in the lives of their friends. They point to the weights of their own babies and to the weights of the babies of friends who smoked and conclude that the scientific evidence must be wrong. Other mothers accept that smoking in pregnancy is harmful yet continue to smoke. They justify their actions by reference to other factors, saying that if they gave up smoking they would become irritable and take it out on the other children or their husbands. They weigh up the risks and decide to safeguard their marriage or the other children hoping that the unborn child will be all right. Some of the mothers were extremely anxious about the subject. Hilary Graham quotes one of them:

> If you must know I'm worried sick about it. I can't stop and there's an end to it. I wish I could just be left alone, my husband goes on, and my mother, and every time I open a magazine I'm told I'm killing my baby, and now it's even on the telly. What're they trying to do?. . . They don't need to tell me, I know I'm harming him, don't they think I've got any feelings and worry myself sick over it?

Health education, like the more general regulations discussed earlier, may be intrusive, and this has led some to suggest that preventive programmes should abandon health education in favour of providing the help that is required by people to alter their lifestyle. Some support for this approach to preventive medicine has been provided by studies in the USA. These have shown that by altering the way in which a service is provided so as to make it acceptable to those for whom it is intended, either behaviour or attitudes may be changed. For instance the Harvard experimental 'comprehensive care program' improved the uptake of vaccine among children, though the mothers' attitudes did not change (Robertson et al, 1974). Lawrence Green (1970) has even suggested that the only attitudes that health professionals have a right to change are those of their fellow professionals. This is an extreme view, but it takes account of the costs that are very often attached to health education, and which are frequently ignored.

Conclusion

Prevention is often better than cure but even preventive programmes have their costs. These include the costs to individuals who enjoy the pleasures of living dangerously, rich food, low residue diets, hang-gliding, smoking, drinking immoderately, staying up late and bicycling, and they also include financial costs, a subject that will be dealt with more fully in Chapter 6.

SECONDARY PREVENTION

The effectiveness of secondary prevention

Secondary prevention is the prevention of the more serious consequences of disease by early diagnosis and treatment. The strategy of secondary prevention requires that the natural history of the disease includes an early phase at which the disease is more easily or more reliably treated. There is also an assumption that a significant proportion of those who have the early disease will progress to the more serious later stages.

In order to justify a secondary prevention programme for a disease it is necessary to have safe and accurate method of detection and a safe and reliable treatment both of which are acceptable to the population at which the programme is aimed. Wilson and Jungner have laid down ten criteria that should be fulfilled before a programme is justified, and these are given in Table 4.4.

Detection of disease within a programme of secondary prevention may be made by screening samples of the general population or groups at special risk and, where necessary, by subsequent referral for a definitive, diagnosis. It may also be made by 'case finding', in which the doctor tests patients who come to the surgery for some other purpose. For instance, as up to 95 per cent of patients who have undiagnosed hypertension have seen the doctor in the previous 5 years, an expensive screening programme may not be necessary for finding the majority of undiagnosed hypertensives if doctors check the blood pressure of all those coming to their surgeries.

Whatever the method of detection, the need for an accurate test is important. A test with poor specificity (Ch. 3) used on large populations will result in a very large number of false positive results. Where the disease being sought is rare there may be many more false positives than true positives. It may be possible to combine the characteristics of two tests in order to exploit first the sensitivity and cheapness of one to find those who are at risk in a large population, and then the specificity of another possibly more expensive test to sift out the true positives from the others. This is

Table 4.4 Criteria for screening programmes (From: Wilson J M G, Jungner G 1968 The principles and practice of screening for disease. WHO PA/66.7.)

1. The condition sought should be an important health problem
2. There should be an accepted treatment for patients with recognised disease
3. Facilities for diagnosis and treatment should be available
4. There should be a recognisable latent or early symptomatic stage
5. There should be a suitable test or examination
6. The test should be acceptable to the population
7. The natural history of the condition, including development from latent to declared disease, should be adequately understood
8. There should be an agreed policy on whom to treat as patients
9. The cost of case-finding (including diagnosis and treatment of patients diagnosed) should be economically balanced in relation to possible expenditure on medical care as a whole
10. Case finding should be a continuing process and not a 'once and for all' project.

done for instance in screening for cancer of the cervix where the cytology from the smear is often followed by a 'cone biopsy' before making a final diagnosis. It is also done in screening for neural tube defects. If the mother's serum alpha-fetoprotein is raised, amniocentesis is generally offered before aborting the fetus.

Many of the treatments offered as secondary prevention have high costs to the patient. To offer these to a patient who is apparently well and generally without any symptoms is not justified unless both the diagnosis is certain and the treatment is efficacious. The use of electronic fetal monitoring during labour has probably contributed to the increase in the number of babies born by Caesarean section. This is clearly a high price for the mothers to pay, though there may be benefits also in terms of reduced perinatal morbidity and mortality. The treatment of breast cancer, cancer of the cervix, and hypertension all have high costs to the patient and to the community, which are only worth paying if the diagnosis is accurate and the treatment efficacious.

Finally, a screening programme, in order to be effective, must reach those who would benefit from it. The incidence of cancer of the cervix continues to rise with age. The majority of new cases occur between the ages of 45 and 65 but the majority of screening examinations occur in the younger age groups, most of them below

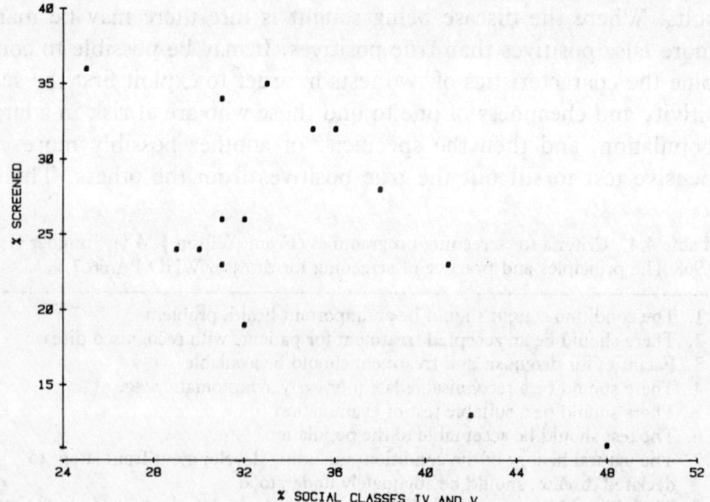

Fig. 4.6 Proportion of women screened for carcinoma of the cervix by proportion of women in social classes IV and V in 15 Oxford wards. (Based on information from: Jackson J 1979 Screening in general practice: cervical cytology for higher risk women. Public Health (London) 93: 300–5.)

the age of 35 when cancer of the cervix is very rare. Moreover, whereas the disease is associated with the poorer sections of the population, the uptake of the screening service is greater in the richer sections. Figure 4.6 shows the uptake of screening for cancer of the cervix in 15 wards of the city of Oxford by the proportion of the population of those wards that is in social classes IV and V.

Multiphasic screening

Multiphasic screening is an extension of the principles of secondary prevention from single diseases to a wide variety of conditions. It is subject to all the problems of the other secondary prevention programmes but on a much larger scale. The number of tests performed make it far more likely that any individual will have a false positive result on one of them, creating a lot of work for the medical services and causing the patient a great deal of unnecessary worry. Generally speaking there are few abnormalities for which there are suitable treatments and which are not already known to the doctor or the patient.

Table 4.5 summarises the results of a randomised trial of a multiphasic screening programme in South East London. In 1967, 6424 people were randomly allocated to two groups. The first group was invited to take part in a screening programme in 1967 and again in 1969; the other group was not invited to the screening programme. Both groups were followed up and studied in 1972. There was no evidence that those who were screened had any better health. They had marginally higher death rates, more hospital admissions, higher

Table 4.5 The effects of multiphasic screening on mortality and morbidity: results of the south-east London Screening Study (From: D'Souza M F 1978 Early diagnosis and multiphasic screening. In: Bennett A E (ed) Recent advances in community medicine. Churchill Livingstone, Edinburgh, pp 195–214.)

	Screened	Controls
Death rates (1967–75) (/1000 man years at risk)	10.0	9.2
Hospital admissions (1967–75) (1000 man years at risk)	50.7	49.6
GP consultation rates (/person/year)		
Men	3.2	3.1
Women	4.0	3.8
% Claiming good or excellent health (in fortnight preceding final survey)	53.2	56.5
% Hypertensive (diastolic B.P. above 104 mmHg)	2.7	3.1

GP consultation rates, and marginally fewer of them claimed that they were in good or excellent health in the two weeks before the final survey. There is very little evidence that multiphasic screening provides any net benefit to the health of the community.

CONCLUSION

The effectiveness of health services is an important attribute, whether these health services are preventive or curative. The characteristics of a service that make it effective include principally the efficacy and safety of the procedures used and the distribution and use made of the service by the population as a whole. The next chapter will discuss the methods used to measure the effectiveness of the health services.

REFERENCES

Ashley J S A, Howlett A, Morris J N 1971 Case fatality of hyperplasia of the prostate in two teaching and three regional-board hospitals. Lancet 2: 1308–11

Belloc N B, Breslow L 1972 Relationship of physical health status and health practices. Preventive Medicine 1: 409–21

Butler J R, Knight R 1975 Designated areas: a review of problems and policies. British Medical Journal 2: 571–3

Davies D M 1977 History and epidemiology. In: Davies D M (ed) Textbook of adverse drug effects. Oxford University Press, Oxford

Fox R H, Woodward P M, Exton-Smith A N, Green M F, Donnison D V, Wicks M H 1973 Body temperature in the elderly: a national study of physiological, social and environmental conditions. British Medical Journal 1: 200–6

Graham H 1976 Smoking in pregnancy: the attitudes of expectant mothers. Social Science and Medicine 10: 399–405

Green L 1970 Should health education abandon attitude change strategies? Health Education Monographs 30: 25–48

Hart J T 1971 The inverse care law. Lancet 2: 1308–11

Knopf A, Wakefield J 1974 Effect of medical education on smoking behaviour. British Journal of Social and Preventive Medicine 28: 246–51

Parkin D 1979 Distance as an influence on demand in general practice. Journal of Epidemiology and Community Health 33: 96–9

Robertson L S, Kosa J, Heaggarty M C, Haggerty R J, Alpert J J 1974 Changing the medical care system: a controlled experiment in comprehensive care. Praeger, New York

FURTHER READING

Professor McKeown was one of the early sceptics who cast doubt on the effectiveness of the health services; his most recent evaluation of their role is to be found in:

McKeown T 1979 The role of medicine: dream mirage or nemesis. Basil Blackwell, Oxford

There are many other followers, but a more optimistic view (sic) of the role of medicine is to be found in:

Dollery C 1978 The end of an age of optimism: medical science in retrospect and prospect. Nuffield Provincial Hospitals Trust

A book that has been very influential in arguing the case for thorough evaluation and which introduced the term effectiveness, though in a slightly different sense, is:

Cochrane A L 1971 Effectiveness and efficiency: random reflections on the health services. Nuffield Provincial Hospitals Trust

A readable introduction to the subject of preventive medicine is:

Gray J A L Muir 1979 Man against disease: preventive medicine. Oxford University Press, Oxford

And a number of authors have contributed to a more specialist volume on health education in:

Sutherland I (ed) 1979 Health education: perspectives and choices. Allen and Unwin, London

5

Assessing efficacy and effectiveness in the health services

INTRODUCTION

The need for evaluation

The careful evaluation of health services is of prime importance. It is sometimes argued that the money spent on evaluation would be better spent on the wider application of the service, the assumption being that the more there is of any service the better it is for the community. But the results of a service until properly evaluated are rarely obvious. Several studies, three of which are described below, have shown that what was, *a priori*, of 'obvious' benefit was in fact of little value.

Supplementing maternal diets

There is adequate evidence that both birth weight and the subsequent mental achievement of a child are related to maternal nutrition during pregnancy. In order to reduce the proportion of low birth weight babies born to a population of poor black women in Harlem, a diet supplementation programme was begun in 1969. The programme was evaluated by a randomised controlled trial, and women were allocated to one of three groups. One group received a 'supplement' to their diet in the form of a drink that they took each day during their pregnancy, the second group received a lesser 'complement' to their diet, and the third group received only the vitamin and iron pills that were given out in the clinics. But the expected benefits of the treatment were not seen as (Table 5.1) there were significantly more neonatal deaths among the babies of the mothers who received the 'supplement'.

Giving iron to the anaemic

It is well known that dietary iron deficiency leads to a hypochromic microcytic anaemia, which generally should be treated with iron supplements. Table 5.2 shows the results of a controlled trial of ferrous sulphate supplement given to Somali nomads entering a re-

Table 5.1 Some results from a trial of nutritional supplementation during pregnancy. (From: Rush D, Stein Z, Susser M 1980 A randomised controlled trial of prenatal nutritional supplementation in New York City. Pediatrics 65: 683–97.)

		Neonatal deaths (number)				
		Gestation at delivery (weeks)				
Treatment group	Births	<28	28–32	32–36	Total	(%)
Supplement	259	4	3	1	8	(3.2)
Complement	270	1	1	1	3	(1.2)
Control	276	2	...	1	3	(1.1)
Total (twins excluded)	805	7	4	3	14	(1.8)

Supplement vs all others $\chi^2 = 4.01, P<.05$
Supplement vs controls $\chi^2 = 2.63$, N.S.

Table 5.2 Some results of treating 'iron depleted' Somali nomads with ferrous sulphate tablets. (From: Murray M J, Murray A B, Murray M, Murray C J 1978 The adverse effect of iron repletion on the course of certain infections. British Medical Journal 2: 1113–5.)

Test	Group	*N*	Before	After	Increase	(%)
Haemaglobin (g/dl)	Treatment	71	8.3	12.3		
	Control	66	8.1	8.7		
Reticulocytes (%)	Treatment	71	0.9	5.1		
	Control	66	0.6	1.2		
Malaria smear (number +ve)	Treatment	71	0	21	21/77	(30)
	Control	66	0	2	2/66	(3)
Parasitaemia (number +ve)	Treatment	71	0	11	11/71	(15)
	Control	66	0	4	4/66	(6)
S. haematobium ova (number +ve)	Treatment	71	3	11	8/71	(11)
	Control	66	2	2	0/66	(0)
Ziehl-Nielsen smear (number +ve)	Treatment	71	0	3	3/71	(4)
	Control	66	0	0	0/66	(0)
Brucella antibody titre > 1:640	Treatment	71	1	14	13/71	(18)
	Control	66	0	0	0/66	(0)
S. typhimurium bacteraemia (number +ve)	Treatment	71	0	6	6/71	(8)
	Control	66	0	0	0/66	(0)

feeding camp in the Ogaden. The nomads given oral iron experienced a reticulocyte response and a rise in haemoglobin levels. However, the treatment cannot be seen as an unqualified success as nomads who received the iron supplement also experienced a rise in the prevalence of malaria, schistosomiasis, tuberculosis, brucellosis and salmonella bacteraemia.

Giving oral hypoglycaemics to maturity onset diabetics

There are a number of drugs that improve the control of blood sugar in non-insulin dependent diabetics. These were seen as a useful aid to the treatment of mature onset diabetes and an improvement on the use of diet alone. In the 1960s the University Group Diabetic Project in America assessed the value of these drugs in a randomised controlled trial. The results of this trial are given in Table 5.3. The mortality among those treated with diet and oral hypoglycaemics appeared higher than that among those treated with diet alone. Although phenformin had always been a drug of last choice as the danger of lactic acidosis was already well documented, the finding that tolbutamide was also disadvantageous was surprising.

Defining success: structure, process and outcome

Evaluative studies can be planned at various levels of complexity. Health services can be evaluated most simply in terms of whether they have the necessary manpower and equipment to perform their tasks. This aspect of health services is known as 'structure'. Measurement of structure is comparatively easy and the results of such studies may be extremely useful in identifying deficiencies. Studies of structure alone, however, give no information on whether the manpower and resources are being put to good use. From this point of view they have serious limitations.

The use made of manpower and other resources is known as 'process'. Measures of process include the number of clinical inves-

Table 5.3 Some results from the University Group Diabetes Program. % dead in 5 years by selected baseline characteristics in the 'UGDP'. (From: The American Diabetes Association 1970 The University Group Diabetes Program. The study of the effects of hypoglycemic agents on vascular complications in patients with adult onset diabetes. Diabetes 19 (Supplement 2): 747–830.)

Cardiovascular risk factors	Treatment			
	Placebo	Tolbutamide	Insulin (fixed dose)	Insulin (variable)
None	2.0	9.0	2.0	0.0
One or more	8.0	15.2	10.9	15.0
Cholesterol >300 mg%	5.9	13.3	14.7	18.5
Hypertension >160/95	6.8	13.3	10.9	19.6
Arterial calcification (right lower limb)	13.6	25.6	25.7	22.6

tigations performed on patients, the number of drugs prescribed, and the number of operations performed. Use of resources is generally well documented, particularly in countries where doctors are paid a fee for service, where the individual patient pays his own medical bills, or where insurance companies pay the bills for the patients. For this reason it is generally possible to measure process, and a large number of process measures have been used to evaluate services. The problem with process is that it may not have any clear relationship to benefits for the patient. It is even possible, as we have already seen, that well intentioned process may actually harm the patient.

'Outcome' is the net benefit from a service to the patients, or to the community. It is a better measure of success than either structure or process. Its major drawback is that information on outcome is hard to obtain without resorting to special surveys. This is not so in some diseases for which there is a high mortality, and where death may be taken as a reasonable measure of outcome; but such diseases are now rare.

Assessing efficacy

The measurement of efficacy is now routine in the assessment of new drugs. The assessment of other procedures is less widespread, partly because it poses greater problems of organisation, partly because of problems in designing adequate trials, and partly, no doubt, because there is not the incentive provided by bodies such as the Committee on the Safety of Medicines and the Food and Drugs Administration.

The evaluation of preventive techniques does not differ greatly from the evaluation of curative procedures. The efficacy of preventive measures may be assessed by comparing the incidence of the disease in those who were not subjected to the procedure (B), with the incidence in those who were subjected to the procedure (A). The efficacy of the procedure can then be computed from the formula:

$$\text{Efficacy} = \frac{(B - A) \times 100\%}{B}$$

This gives a value of 100 per cent if no cases occur in the experimental group (A), and 0 per cent if the procedure is worthless.

The efficacy of preventive strategies tends, however, to be more difficult to evaluate than that of curative techniques because it is more difficult to keep cases and controls separate. Two examples will clarify this point. Where a large proportion of the population is immunised against an epidemic disease, herd immunity will protect the unimmunised. Any study within such a population will therefore underestimate the efficacy of the vaccine, because even the unimmunised will benefit from the herd immunity conferred on them by those who have been immunised. The second example is from the evaluation of a health education programme in northern Finland where there was a major attempt to reduce the amount of heart disease. A massive programme was mounted to persuade people to reduce their fat intake, to have their blood pressure checked and treated if it was found to be raised, and to give up smoking. In evaluating the results of this study (Puska et al, 1979) it was noted that the prevalence of these three risk factors had declined both in North Karelia, where the programme had taken place, and in other parts of Finland as well. It is possible that the decline in the prevalence of risk factors in other parts of Finland was also partly due to the health education programme in North Karelia. If this was the case the actual results of the study underestimate the effects of the health education programme.

Assessing effectiveness

Whereas efficacy is a characteristic of procedures applied to individuals, effectiveness is a characteristic of services offered to communities. For this reason in a trial of efficacy it is the individual patient who is allocated to the treatment or control group; in a trial of effectiveness it is groups of people, communities, villages, practices or clinic catchment areas that are allocated. These are the units of observation, rather than individuals, and the analysis will be a comparison of the prevalence or incidence of problems in these units.

These larger units of observation raise a number of problems. First, any study of effectiveness will inevitably be large, for there must be enough units of observation to make it unlikely that any difference between the 'experimental' and 'control' groups is due to chance. The more variation that there is between the units at the beginning of the study, the larger the trial will have to be. For this reason full experimental studies on the effectiveness of different policies are rare.

Second, the constitution of these units may be changing. Particularly in trials of effectiveness which take a long time there may not only be births and deaths, but also migration in and out of the units. As the characteristics of migrants are different from those who stay behind, over the long periods required to test the effectiveness of some health care procedures, this may have a considerable effect on the results.

Sometimes the units are too large for an experimental study and some other type of study must be performed. There are some interventions, for instance the compulsory use of seatbelts, that are only introduced by national or state legislation. It is not possible to randomise countries or states into those which will and those which will not introduce legislation of this kind. Each country will decide its own policy independently, and it is not practical to expect local experiments which would require the law to vary at random from the national, state or provincial legislation. In such cases some other experimental design must be used.

Assessing acceptability

Any evaluation must be based on assumptions about what is valuable. In medicine this means principally what is valuable to the patient. Assumptions often have to be made about this, but these ought to be examined critically, as they are frequently misjudged.

We can see two examples of this if we look at the concept of survival time. The outcome of a disease with a high mortality is often assessed by computing the proportion of patients alive 5 years after diagnosis, or 5 years after treatment. A number of criticisms have been levelled against this rather crude measure, and, to illustrate one such criticism the proportion surviving after two different treatments for chronic renal failure are given in Figure 5.1. Slightly

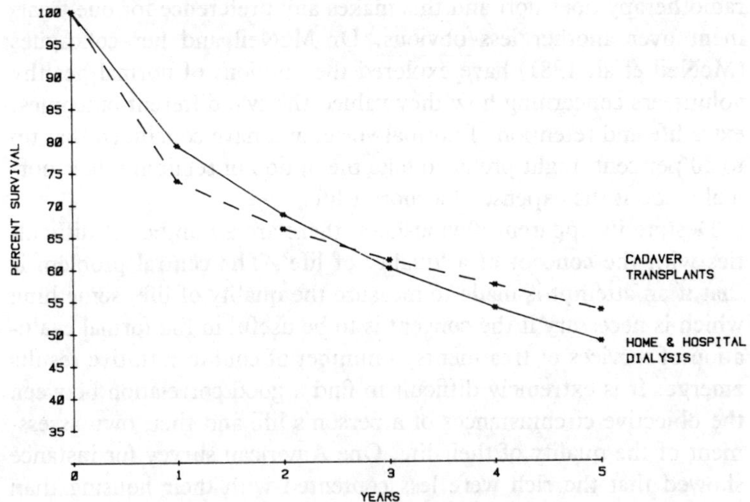

Fig. 5.1 Survival curves for patients aged 45–54 years with chronic renal failure for two different treatments. (From data supplied by the European Dialysis and Transplant Association.)

more of those receiving surgery were alive at 5 years, compared with those on dialysis, and it might be concluded that surgery was therefore the treatment of choice. But closer inspection of the graph shows that this increased survival at 5 years is bought at the cost of a higher expectation of being dead at 1 year. A similar result has been found comparing treatments for a number of other conditions, and McNeil and her colleagues (1978) have discussed the options for patients with lung cancer. Here again surgery has a better long term, but a worse short term prognosis. These authors have explored some of the implications of this. They have suggested that some people put a relatively higher value on immediate survival than on the long term result and that, where this is so, the conventional measure of success, 5 year survival, is inappropriate. The central point is that no single course of action is axiomatic, and that apparently neutral assessments of outcome may hide a number of value judgements.

Survival must also be matched against the quality of life. The price that has to be paid for an extra year or so of life may well be more than the patient regards as acceptable. For instance, there are two recognised treatments available for the treatment of carcinoma of the larynx, surgery and radiotherapy. For stage T3 carcinoma of the larynx the 3 year survival following surgery is estimated at 60 per cent, whereas for radiotherapy it is only 30–40 per cent. On the other hand surgery leads to a loss of normal speech whereas radiotherapy does not, and this makes any preference for one treatment over another less obvious. Dr McNeil and her colleagues (McNeil et al, 1981) have explored the opinions of normal healthy volunteers concerning how they valued the two different outcomes, extra life and retention of normal voice, and have concluded that up to 20 per cent might prefer to take the option of retaining their normal voice at the expense of a shorter life.

Despite its apparent obviousness, there are a number of difficulties with the concept of a 'quality of life'. The central problem is that if an attempt is made to measure the quality of life, something which is necessary if the concept is to be useful in the formal evaluation of services or treatments, a number of counterintuitive results emerge. It is extremely difficult to find a good correlation between the objective circumstances of a person's life and their own assessment of the quality of their life. One American survey for instance showed that the rich were less contented with their housing than the poor, who had objectively less satisfactory housing. The discrepancy arises in part because our perceptions of our lives depend to a large extent on our expectations; our perceptions of various aspects of our lives, such as our housing or health, depend on other unrelated circumstances, such as the closeness of our family and friends. Satisfaction with treatment received has also been shown to depend on the amount of information that a patient receives about his treatment, a factor that some doctors might regard as not altogether relevant to some particular treatment.

The difficulties of assessing the acceptability or the effect of a treatment on the quality of life are great enough when dealing with just the individual patient. They are even greater when the concepts have to be applied to populations. In this case it is not the problem faced by an individual patient who has to chose between two imperfect solutions. A choice may have to be made between the good of two groups of patients, for instance between investing in a bone marrow transplant centre or in new accommodation for the elderly. More will be said of this particular problem in the next chapter.

STUDY DESIGN

The evaluation of health services takes place at different levels of sophistication. The same criteria and the same thoroughness of design are not suitable under all circumstances. The most thorough studies are those that are generally conducted when a new technique is introduced. These are now most often randomised controlled trials and will be discussed in some detail as they tend to be the model against which other methods are compared.

The formal assessment of a technique may be required where randomisation is not possible, particularly when the technique is already established. Under these circumstances there are a number of other designs that can be used though they are in some ways less satisfactory. Simple designs are also used when collecting information for managers or clinicians to monitor the performance of the service. In these circumstances rigour is sacrificed for simplicity, and the results must be interpreted with caution.

The randomised controlled trial

Figure 5.2 illustrates the design of a randomised controlled trial. The basic idea is that those who might benefit from the new treatment are divided into two groups which are, as far as possible, similar to each other in every respect. One group then receives the new treatment, and the other group receives either the established

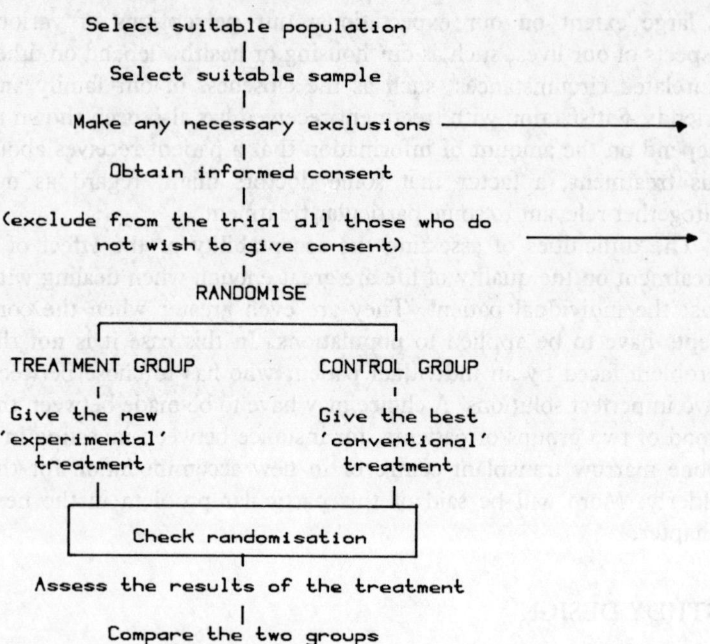

Fig. 5.2 Design of a randomised controlled trial.

treatment for the complaint or, if there is none, a placebo, a treatment that is known to be pharmacologically inactive. The results of the treatment for the two groups are then compared.

Defining the relevant group, and choosing a sample

The first task is to define the groups of patients who are eligible for the trial. Cases who would not benefit or might be harmed by the new treatment must be excluded in advance because, once the trial has begun, every individual who presents for the trial and is not specifically excluded must be entered. If it is subsequently decided that they should not receive one of the treatments prescribed by the trial, they must still count as part of the group to which they have been randomised. This must be so to avoid bias in selecting 'suitable' patients for one or other group.

When the criteria for inclusion and exclusion have been decided a group of eligible patients has to be found. These are usually patients attending a particular hospital department or general practice. This is necessary for practical reasons, but it must be established that there is nothing peculiar about the group that makes them unrepresentative of the wider group of patients for whom the treatment will eventually be used.

Random allocation

Before entering the trial, the patients' eligibility should be checked and their informed consent obtained. The patients are then entered into the trial at random either into the experimental group or into the control group. The random allocation implies that any individual has an equal chance of being entered into either group. It is not enough to enter alternate patients into each group, or to enter patients with certain initials into different groups, for either of these systems may bias the results if the order in which the patients arrive is not itself random, or if there is some non-random element in the allocation of initials, the Mc's, for instance, being dominated by the Scots. The correct method of randomisation has been discussed more fully in Chapter 3.

Random allocation has a number of advantages. Statistical theory allows us to predict that, given a large number of patients in each group, their characteristics, as groups, will be similar. This similarity will apply not only to characteristics that are known to be likely to affect the results but also to characteristics of which we are unaware, but which may still be important. It also allows the general assumption that, even if characteristics believed to be important cannot be measured, they will have a known probability of being equally distributed between the two groups. Sometimes the groups of patients are so small that it is not reasonable to assume that they will contain similar characteristics by chance. This can be partially overcome by stratifying. If it is known that one or two factors are particularly likely to influence the outcome, the patients can first be grouped into 'strata' according to these characteristics and then the members of each stratum equally divided at random between those who receive the treatment and the controls. This ensures that patients with certain known prognostic indicators are allocated randomly but equally between the two groups.

When a new technique is first introduced it is often argued that the technique is so obviously good that such random allocation is unacceptable, and that historical rather than contemporary controls should be used. This means that the current group of patients receiving the new treatment are compared with patients who were treated with the old treatment in the past. This is almost never satisfactory because patients from the past are unlikely to be similar in all respects to patients being treated now except the new treatment. There may, for instance, be a trend for patients to present earlier in the course of the disease; if this is so the cases who presented later in the disease (the historical controls) will appear to have died earlier even if the time from the onset of the disease to

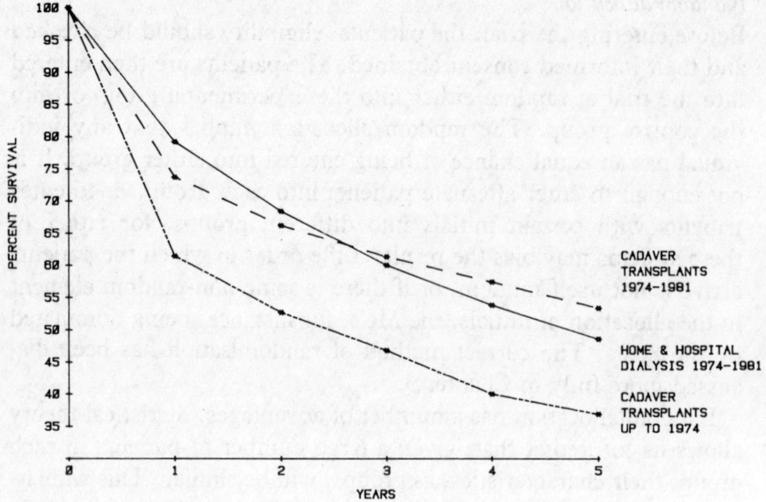

Fig. 5.3 Survival curves for patients aged 45–54 years with chronic renal failure for two treatments and for two periods of time. (From data supplied by the European Dialysis and Transplant Association.)

death is the same in each group. The methods of assessing patients also change, so that it may be hard to tell whether like is being compared with like. Furthermore the other services that patients receive become more sophisticated.

Figure 5.3 shows the survival of patients aged 45–54 with chronic renal failure according to the treatment they received. Two curves are the same as those shown in Figure 5.1 and show the results for patients with cadaver transplants and on haemodialysis in the period 1974–81. The patients who received the cadaver transplants did slightly better than the haemodialysis patients at 5 years. For comparison we have added the survival curve for those receiving cadaver transplants in the period before 1974. This group did worse than either of the other two groups. If a trial had been done to compare the two types of treatment comparing haemodialysis patients in the latter period with historical controls who had received cadaver transplants the wrong conclusions would have been drawn.

Follow-up

The patients must be followed up. This may be over a very short period, or for many years. The observations on which the success or failure of the trial will be judged must be determined in advance of the trial and made in a standard way to minimise error. To minimise bias in these measurements and to prevent patients being given treatment other than according to the protocol, it is wise to ensure that neither patient nor doctor knows which treatment is being given. When the patient does not know, the trial is described as single blind; when neither knows the trial is double blind.

Analysis

Although there are techniques which allow for the analysis of the data as they are collected ('sequential analysis') it is more usual to analyse the results at the end of the trial when all the information has been collected. At this stage it is important that all the individuals who entered the trial are accounted for. It is not permissible, for instance, to exclude those who did not comply with the treatment; and every effort must be made to find out what happened to those who have dropped out of the trial for one reason or another. Table 5.4 shows the results from a trial of the drug clofibrate. Those who complied with the treatment, whether this was

Table 5.4 Relationship between adherence and mortality in a drug trial. (From: The Coronary Drug Project Research Group 1980 Influence of adherence to treatment and response of cholesterol on mortality in the coronary drug project. New England Journal of Medicine 303: 1038–41.)

	Treatment Clofibrate		Placebo	
Adherence	Number of patients	% Mortality + s.e. (adjusted %)	Number of patients	% Mortality + s.e. (adjusted %)
< 80%	357	24.6 + 2.3 (22.5)	882	28.2 + 1.5 (25.8)
> 80% =	708	15.0 + 1.3 (15.7)	1813	15.1 + 0.8 (16.4)
Total	1065	18.2 + 1.2 (18.0)	2695	19.4 + 0.8 (19.5)

clofibrate or placebo, had a lower mortality than those who failed to comply. The overall mortality is however similar for the two groups. If those who had failed to take the clofibrate had been excluded from the trial the results would have been biased and would have shown quite erroneously that clofibrate was superior to a placebo. The exclusion of drop-outs from the analysis may seriously bias the results of a trial.

Objections to randomised controlled trials

Two general objections to randomised controlled trials are often put forward: that they are unethical, and that randomisation is impractical.

Ethical objections

The first objection to randomised controlled trials is that they are unethical because a group of patients is being offered a treatment that is known to be ineffective, or at least less effective than the best treatment known. Occasionally this objection is justified. There was no randomised trial of streptomycin in the treatment of miliary tuberculosis which, before streptomycin, was universally and rapidly fatal and no trial was required: but this situation is rare. More often the efficacy of the treatment is in doubt, and the possible side-effects unknown. A number of cases have already been cited where what appeared to be a sensible treatment proved to be deleterious to the patients when properly assessed.

If no adequate randomised trial is performed at the introduction of a new technique, it becomes increasingly difficult to perform one. Early on there is rarely enough of a new technology to go round, and it is therefore inevitable that some patients will have to go without. There can therefore be no ethical problem in withholding the new treatment from some. On the contrary, during the development of a new treatment it is ethically preferable to offer or withhold the new treatment at random as both the long term side effects and the efficacy in human subjects are still unknown. It is not reasonable to subject a group of patients to the new treatment as if it were of known benefit without these aspects being fully investigated. In the study of clofibrate, the drug did reduce cholesterol levels in those who took it, and there was a reduction in the mortality from heart disease. The treatment failed because there was at the same time a rise in the death rate from other diseases among those on clofibrate. This could not have been predicted before the trial.

However, anxieties do remain in the minds of both clinicians and patients concerning the ethical standing of randomised trials. An alternative has been suggested by Zelen (1979), which is illustrated in Figure 5.4. In this the patients are randomised into two groups as in the traditional randomised controlled trial. The control group is given the standard treatment, again as in the classical trial. The difference is in the treatment group. These patients are not given the new treatment automatically but are offered a choice between the new treatment and the standard treatment. The results of all of

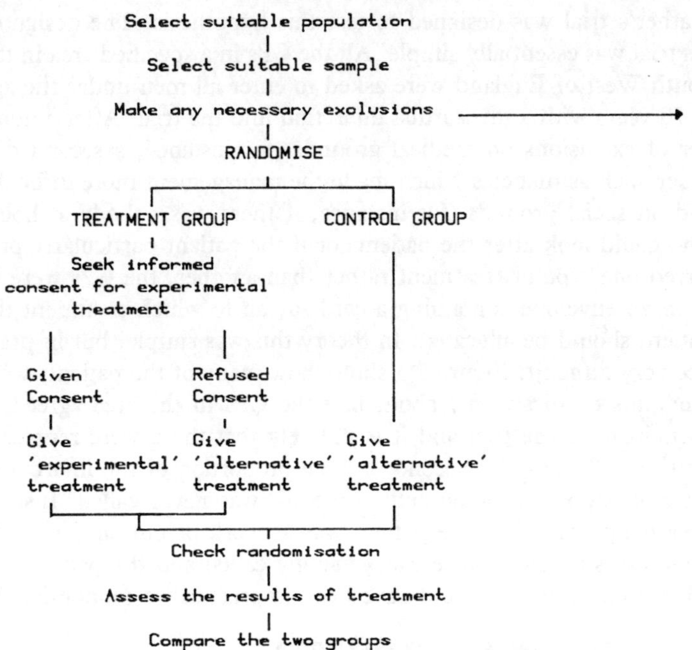

Fig. 5.4 Zelen's modified design for a randomised controlled trial. (Adapted from: Zelen M 1979 A new design for randomised clinical trials. New England Journal of Medicine 300: 1242–5.)

those randomised to each group, regardless of which treatment they received, are then compared. The advantage of this design is that the clinician does not appear to his patients to be acting in an arbitrary way. The disadvantage is that the treatment group is diluted with patients who are receiving the same treatment as the controls. This will make any difference between the two treatments more difficult to detect. It is too early to comment on the success of this design as there is little experience of it. Its success will largely depend on how many of those randomised to the treatment group volunteer to take the new treatment.

Practical objections

The practical objections to randomised controlled trials can be illustrated by Mather's trial of home versus hospital treatment of men with myocardial infarction. It had been noted that the survival rate among men with infarcts was about equal among men admitted to hospital coronary care units, and among men treated at home by their GPs. It was possible to interpret this finding by suggesting that those admitted to hospital were the more severe cases.

Mather's trial was designed to test this hypothesis. The design of his trial was essentially simple. All the GPs in a specified area in the South West of England were asked to enter all men under the age of 70 years with a myocardial infarction into the trial. After a number of exclusions on medical grounds (for instance, a second disorder such as diabetes which made the management more difficult) and on social grounds (for instance, if there was nobody at home who could look after the patient) or if the patient particularly preferred one type of treatment rather than another, the GPs were to open an envelope containing a card saying to which treatment the patient should be allocated. In theory this was simple, but in practice very difficult. Figure 5.5 shows how many of the patients were randomised. First, only about half the GPs in the area agreed to participate in the trial and it is unlikely that these were representative of all the GPs. Second, a large proportion of the infarctions did not happen at home and so the GP was never called. Instead they happened when the patient was at work or out shopping. In these cases an ambulance was generally called and the patient was taken to hospital; it would have been impractical to randomise the

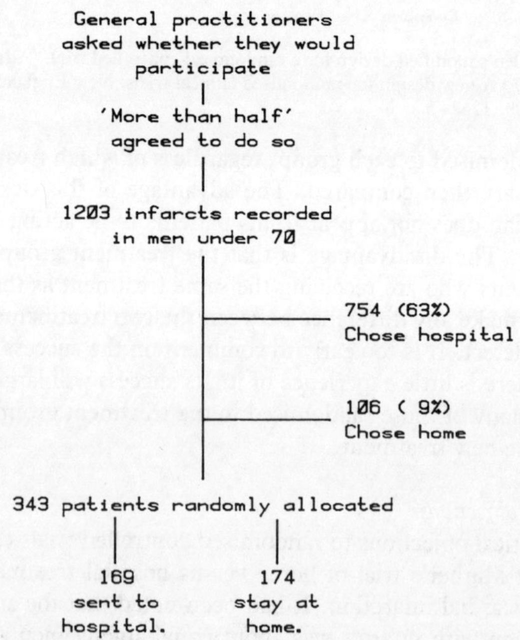

Fig. 5.5 The randomisation of patients in Mather's trial of home vs hospital treatment of acute myocardial infarction. (From information in: Mather H G, Pearson N G, Read K L Q et al 1971 Acute myocardial infarction: home vs hospital treatment. British Medical Journal 3: 334–8.)

patients back into the care of their GPs once they had arrived in hospital. Third, some of the patients who had infarcts at home called the emergency service instead of the GP; these patients also went to hospital before they could enter the trial. Finally there were all the patients who had been excluded from the trial by the conditions laid down in advance. The trial showed no difference between those treated at home and those treated in hospital.

Such restrictions on randomisation impose limitations on the way that the data can be interpreted. The results refer to the patients of GPs who were willing to take responsibility for their patients under these circumstances; the same results may not have been found if all GPs had been forced to care for their patients, as would be the case if the hospitals made it difficult for GPs to admit these patients. It also refers only to those who had their infarction at home and who called the doctor rather than an ambulance. It might be that if a patient has to be moved he will do better in a coronary care unit and that it is only those who are not moved who will do as well at home.

The practical objections to randomised controlled trials become greater as the form of treatment becomes more complex. But where a randomised controlled trial is truely impractical it should be borne in mind that no other form of experiment will provide the same assurance that bias has been eliminated.

OTHER STUDY DESIGNS

Because it is not always possible to perform a randomised controlled trial it is sometimes necessary to use another type of study to assess the effectiveness of a service. These alternative designs do not provide such good information as the randomised controlled trial, but they may nevertheless provide useful results. Some of the more commonly used designs will be discussed here, with some of their disadvantages.

Post-test static group comparison

In these studies a group which has undergone a procedure is compared with another group which has not. The study is known as a post-test comparison because no measurements are made before the intervention. Before the study that Mather undertook on the effects of home treatment for patients with myocardial infarction, a post-test static group comparison had shown that those who had entered hospital had done no better than those who had stayed at home. This study was useful because it questioned the assumption that those going to hospital would be bound to do better. However, there were several other possible explanations for the result. It might have been that the patients who went to the hospital were sicker in the first place than those who stayed at home. Only the randomised controlled trial settled this issue.

Pre-test/post-test static group comparison

In order to check on the similarity between the two groups being compared after the intervention, it is sometimes possible to obtain information on the state of the patients before the intervention took place. If this is done for both those who received the treatment and for those who did not it is known as a pre-test/post-test static group comparison. Jennet used this design to study the effects of treatment for severe head injury. Because the condition is one with an overall poor outcome, and because it occurs frequently in young people there is a strong compulsion to do as much as is possible to help. For this reason it was impossible to perform a randomised controlled trial of the currently used treatments, and an observational study was planned and implemented in three cities, Glasgow, Rotterdam and Los Angeles. Before treatment, the patients were assessed according to a common protocol which included the depth of the coma, the reactions of the pupils, the presence of haematoma as well as the age of the patient. The different methods of intervention were noted and the outcome was recorded as the percentage of patients who were dead or vegetative at 6 months. Table 5.5 shows some of the results of this study. The number of patients who were dead at 6 months was larger than expected in the group who received steroids, in the group that were ventilated and in the group who had a trachaeostomy. The excess of deaths in the group who were ventilated was statistically significant.

Jennet has discussed at some length the possible explanations for this finding. First it is possible that intervention is more dangerous

Table 5.5 The effect of treatment on the outcome of severe head injury. The expected outcome has been estimated allowing for the age, depth of coma, pupil reaction, presence of haematoma and the country of treatment. (From: Jennet B et al 1980 Treatment for severe head injury. Journal of Neurology, Neurosurgery, and Psychiatry 43: 289–95.)

Therapy	Number of deaths			
	Without this therapy		With this therapy	
	Expected	Observed	Expected	Observed
Steroids	232.4	232	193.6	194
Ventilation	274.9	249	152.1	178
Trachaeostomy	320.2	319	106.8	108

than restraint. On the other hand the study was not a randomised trial and it is possible that there were other factors that led the doctors in charge of the cases to intervene which were not recorded on the protocol. If this is so it may well be that the patients who were less well in the first place were still more often assigned to the more drastic treatment, and that this is not allowed for by simply taking into account the few variables that were recorded in the protocol. This explanation is not considered very probable and it is at least reasonable on the strength of Jennet's study, to perform a formal randomised trial.

Time series analysis

Sometimes it is not possible to have a comparison group, but there are a number of observations that have been made both before and after the intervention which can be analysed for a change in trend. Figure 5.6 shows the notifications for whooping-cough in England and Wales around the time of introduction of the whooping-cough vaccine. This downward trend attracted a great deal of controversy, some saying that it showed that the vaccine had been effective, and some arguing that it merely showed a continuation of a trend that had already been well established before the introduction of the vaccine. The trend after the fall in the uptake of the vaccine was

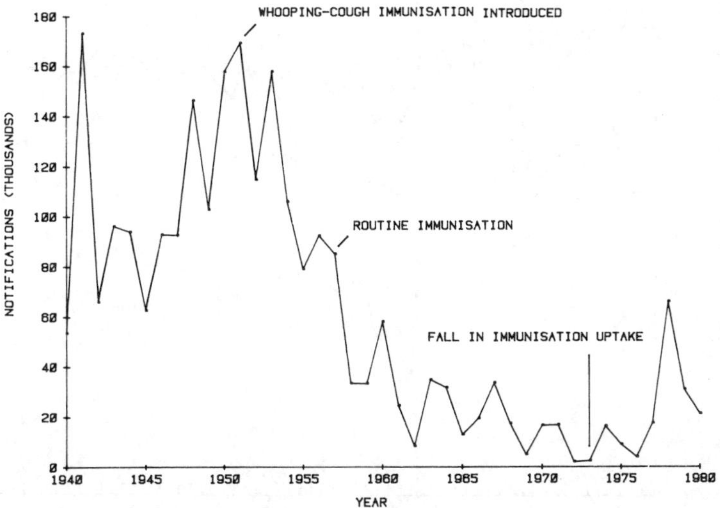

Fig. 5.6 Notifications of whooping-cough in England and Wales, 1940–80. (From data given in: Department of Health and Social Security 1981 Whooping cough: report from the Committee on Safety of Medicines and the Joint Committee on Vaccination and Immunisastion. HMSO, London.)

less ambiguously in favour of the theory that the vaccine was effective. The main problem with time series analysis is the difficulty in distinguishing the effect of the intervention from the effect of other extraneous factors, or, in the case of a single disease, from the effect of time.

Sometimes it is possible to analyse multiple time series in such a way as to give more information. A variation on this technique is shown in Figure 5.7. The number of fatal motor vehicle accidents was recorded before and after the introduction of the breathalyser test. It can be seen that the introduction of the test was followed by a rapid fall in the number of fatal accidents at weekends. The same trend is not seen in the statistics for fatal accidents at other times of the week. It is possible to argue that as the prevalence of drunken driving is higher at the weekends, this supports the contention that the fall in accidents is due to the introduction of the breathalyser test.

SURVEILLANCE AND AUDIT

Apart from experimental trials and other *ad hoc* studies to investigate particular aspects of the health services, there is a need for

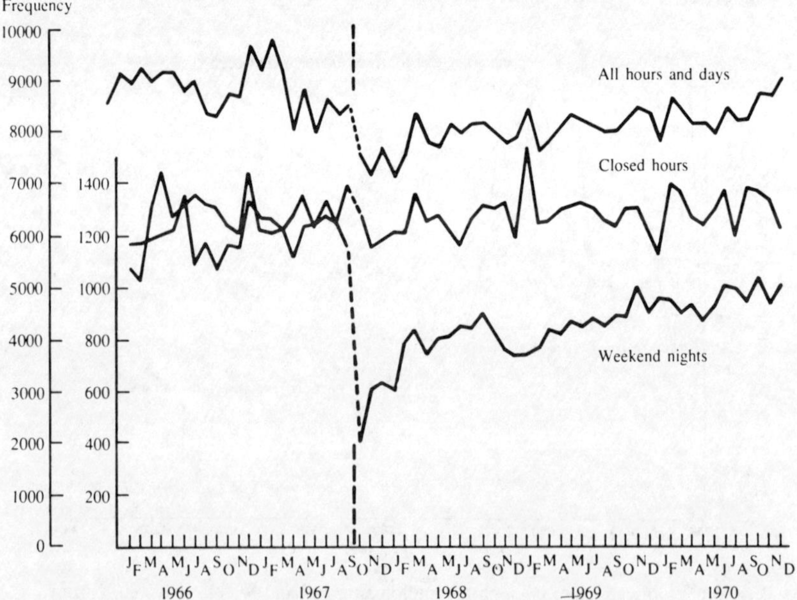

Fig. 5.7 British road casualties before and after the introduction of the breathalyser in October 1967. (Reproduced from: Campbell D T, Cook T D 1978 Quasi-experimentation: Design and analysis for field settings. Houghton Mifflin. With kind permission of the authors.)

simpler methods to review their performance on a continuous basis. The formality of the system that does this varies a great deal; we have divided the methods somewhat arbitrarily into surveillance methods and audit.

Monitoring means the routine collection of information on health, or on the performance of the health services, and in Britain dates in its present form from the middle of the last century. Information is routinely collected and published on discharges from hospital, deaths, infectious diseases, abortions, births and congenital abnormalities, air pollution, inspections carried out by the school medical service, as well as other aspects of health service performance. This information is used in *ad hoc* studies.

Surveillance implies rather more than monitoring, though the difference is greater in theory than practice. It implies that there is a specific objective for the collection of the data, that there is a prearranged point at which the health services or some other agency such as the welfare services or the education services will intervene, and that the form of the intervention is at least in principle also decided in advance, Surveillance systems in this sense are rare. They require a very clear idea not only of what changes would be significant, but also of what sort of action would be required to improve the situation. In addition they require specific information which is often difficult to collect accurately, and which, if it is specific to one surveillance system, may be very expensive to collect for the small returns that could be expected.

Audit implies a method of quality control on a smaller scale. It may be an external audit in which the practice of some part of the service is assessed by outside observers, or, more commonly, it may be an internal audit in which a group of doctors review their own practice. The methods used vary. There may be inquiries into deaths, such as the maternal mortality inquiry, and the increasingly popular perinatal death inquiries. These amount to a full discussion of the management of the patients and some assessment of whether there were any 'avoidable factors'. They tend to be clinically oriented and are based on the consensus judgement of fellow professionals, rather than on the formal epidemiological assessment of the deaths. They are flexible and make a major contribution to continuing medical education. Conducted in the right atmosphere they are not, or should not be, too harrowing an experience for the professionals concerned.

At the other end of the spectrum there are more formal methods of audit that concentrate on the process of care rather than on outcome. The doctors involved in the schemes agree on what constitutes 'good practice' in the care of certain conditions. These criteria are then used to monitor the actual practice of the doctors. These schemes seem to have an effect in that they encourage the good practice that the doctors have agreed, but whether they have any effect on the outcome of the patients is disputed. They may not even improve overall patient care if they encourage the doctor to perform some tests which are unwarranted for a particular patient, merely to avoid censure by arbitrary criteria relevant only to the 'general' case.

CONCLUSION

This chapter has reviewed some of the methods that are used to assess the performance of the health services. The efficacy, the effectiveness and the acceptability of the health services and their procedures are however only one side of the equation. The next chapter will discuss how it is possible to put a price on these options and to decide on which should be provided.

REFERENCES

McNeil B J, Weichselbaum R, Pauker S G 1978 Fallacy of the five year survival in lung cancer. New England Journal of Medicine 299: 1397–401

McNeil B J, Weichselbaum R, Pauker S G 1981 Speech and survival: tradeoffs between quality and quantity of life in laryngeal cancer. New England Journal of Medicine 305: 982–7

Puska P, Salonen J, Tuomilheto J et al 1979 Changes in coronary risk factors during comprehensive five-year community programme to control cardiovascular diseases (North Karelia project). British Medical Journal 2: 1173–8

FURTHER READING

Most textbooks of epidemiology contain chapters on methods of evaluation. The most accessible of these are:

Barker D J P, Rose G 1979 Epidemiology in medical practice. Churchill Livingstone, Edinburgh

Alderson M 1976 An introduction to epidemiology. Macmillan, London

Clinical trials are covered in:

Johnson F N, Johnson S (eds) 1977 Clinical trials. Blackwell Scientific, Oxford

There is a moderately short introduction to the more complex issues of evaluating health services in the American text:

Shortell S, Richardson W C 1978 Health program evaluation. CV Mosby, St Louis

The use of routinely collected information to monitor the health services is discussed in a simple and practical English book:

Tyrrell M 1975 Using numbers for effective Health Service Management. Heinemann Medical, London

Finally, the subject of audit, in the widest sense, is discussed in a collection of distinguised contributions from people working in a wide variety of capacities within the health services:

McLachlan G (ed) 1976 A question of quality? Roads to assurance in medical care. Oxford University Press, Oxford

6

Choosing options

In the last chapter we examined a number of courses of action which contribute to the health of the community. This chapter presents the fundamental reasons why a choice must frequently be made between options for action and the criteria used for such choices.

The central reason for making a choice between alternative methods of improving community health is the impossibility of pursuing every method in full. Health services currently account for between 5.5 and 9.5 per cent of developed countries' national incomes and a detailed reckoning of public health measures (water supply, sewage disposal etc.) would take this figure still higher. To continue all these programmes and to add all schemes of possible benefit would take expenditure beyond the levels acceptable to the electorate. People do not care about their health to the exclusion of all other wants or desires—they may even knowingly damage their health in pursuit of other desires—and so health programmes are inevitably restrained by the community's willingness to pay for them. Reconciling options with resources is an economic decision.

Economics, although associated by the general public with the world of business, banking and money, is essentially concerned with the choice between alternative uses of a fixed budget or fixed manpower. The guiding, and perhaps obvious, principle of economics is 'If you cannot do everything, do the maximum possible'. Within a given cost budget, the preferred programmes will be those which lead to the maximum benefit. However, before examining the criteria on which choices are made, we need to consider who is to make the choice.

WHO IS TO CHOOSE?

Much of economics and economic activity is centred on individuals who make their own choice between alternative uses of their time and money. It is by responding to these choices that the market system operates. However, in the case of health options in Britain, much of the power to choose lies with the government rather than the individual. The individual's choice is restricted to periodic visits to a polling booth.

At least four separate arguments underpin the involvement of government in choosing health options. These can be characterised as the 'externality' defence, the 'paternalistic' defence, the 'redistributive' defence and the 'monopoly' defence.

Externalities

The externality defence, covering air pollution and vaccination programmes, among others, refers to areas of action where individual choice would have an effect on others who are external in the sense that they are not consulted in the individual's choice. Consider first air pollution. If a man burns coal, his neighbours have to put up with the smoke. It may affect their health or their washing. Either way, they are not part of his decision to buy and burn coal. Similarly, if he chooses not to have a preventive vaccination then the neighbourhood may face a higher risk of infection but, again, the neighbours are not a part of the decision to buy or decline the vaccination. External effects of this kind are best resolved by turning them into internal effects. In plain language, the neighbours can enter the decision-making by forcing him to see the effect on them and act accordingly or by giving him an incentive to act in their interests.

In the case of air pollution, either solution is possible. Society as a whole can enforce desirable outcome by legislation, as it has in the Clean Air Act. Alternatively, commodities such as coal which cause pollution could be heavily taxed to encourage the use of a cheaper, smokeless fuel. In the case of vaccination, liberal democracies are usually unhappy with compulsory medication and so the use of incentives will often be preferred to legislation. Free provision of vaccinations results in a high up-take but there is no particular reason, if the benefits of increased herd immunity are large, why cash payments should not be added as a further incentive. Benefits in cash or kind have been used in some birth control programmes in developing countries, where the effect of an extra birth is to put further strain on food supplies and public services.

Governments are, of course, no more than the representatives of the people. The solutions to some problems of external effects could be achieved by small groups of people without the need for government. For example, a committee may be able to decide on rules for cigarette smoking that take account of the external effects of smoke on non-smokers. However, for many external problems, notably those associated with pollution, local action by a small group is ineffective. Hence, national or local government provides a more effective mechanism for achieving a solution than some new assembly of interested parties, not least because it already has the means to raise the money to finance any expenditure or to enforce new legislation.

In every developed country, income support or health services are provided for the chronic sick who cannot provide for themselves. This has led to a widening of the externality argument, beyond its initial associations with environmental health. If one man burns coal or catches an infectious disease his neighbour may be affected. Therefore, he is forced to burn coke and encouraged to receive a free injection by the government to protect his neighbour. However, if he falls ill due to his own behaviour, and can no longer pull his weight in the economy, his neighbour is again affected, as a taxpayer, by the government's commitment to bear the costs of the care provided. Therefore, the argument runs, the government should protect taxpayers against the 'misbehaviour' of others.

Cigarette smoking is an area of behaviour where the externality argument is frequently encountered. Smokers are alleged to be a burden because the community bears the cost of illnesses brought on by smoking. It is possible that in certain circumstances the smoking of cigarettes does impose a burden on the rest of society. However, a careful assessment is required before it can be concluded that smokers are a burden on the rest of society. Smokers pay heavily for their pleasure through high taxes, and also die earlier. The consequence of their premature end and the health services they receive, compared to those received by a healthy non-smoker who lives to an age where permanent care is required, is that they may draw less from health and social security budgets than they contribute (Atkinson & Meade, 1974; Atkinson & Townsend, 1977).

None of this denies the logic of some externality arguments concerning personal behaviour. Individuals who refuse to wear seat-belts when driving pay no extra taxes, yet their injuries impose an appreciable burden on health services funded by others. The difficulty with the argument here is that all relevant activities may not be identifiable. Why should one man's wish not to wear a seatbelt be overriden by government when his neighbour's wish to work too hard, causing stress-related illness to himself and his family, is not open to government control?

Paternalism

Public action to override individual choice in areas of personal life which cannot be shown, on balance, to be damaging to the rest of society, must be viewed as paternalistic. Essentially, the government takes the view that it knows better than the individual what is good for him. The choices made on behalf of children are, by definition, paternalistic. Similarly, the choice made for motorcyclists to wear helmets is a paternalistic one, regardless of the age of the motorcyclist. Essentially, it is being argued that no rational person would choose to exchange the safety of the helmet for the pleasure of unencumbered motoring. As with children and the insane, the individual is protected from his own irrationality. The most plausible explanation of the imposition of helmets upon motorcyclists is that they are a minority group without the political influence of the motoring lobby.

Progress towards the compulsory introduction of other protective measures, such as the use of seatbelts and the fluoridation of water supplies has been much slower, in the face of considerable public disquiet. However, we should not overlook a further feature of the question, the possibility of harm being done by the protective policy. Objections to the compulsory use of seatbelts are often based on the alleged harmful effects, to people trapped in burning cars for example. Similarly, objections to compulsory fluoridation derive from claims that fluoridation would cause other diseases in susceptible individuals. In these cases, compulsion would at times impose additional harm, or so it is claimed, and therefore would constitute an unacceptable imposition on those affected. A debate of the kind that has surrounded these two health options may not be readily resolved. The argument hinges on hypothetical circumstances quite often and so evidence from epidemiological research may not fully resolve some doubts. On the other hand, a growing body of evidence from other locations may contribute to a weakening of the opposition to the measures, leading to their gradual acceptance.

Paternalism also underlies the health service policies of most Western European countries. These countries typically require individuals to make some provision for their health care. In Britain, taxes to finance the NHS are compulsory. In the rest of Europe, public or private health insurance is compulsory to ensure that individuals, through their own choice, are not left without health care. The element of compulsion is designed to protect the individual from his own short-sightedness in purchasing health insurance. Failure to appreciate that one day he may need it could lead the healthy individual to ignore health insurance. When he does need it, the state will bear the burden, for philanthropic reasons, and so the state in turn tries to reduce the size of this burden by legislation. The burden of health care costs comes particularly from the old yet they are the group with least income to pay their own way. Thus, governments may intervene to ensure that adequate provision is made for the old through taxation. A similar argument applies to pensions. In both fields it is assumed that the individual would be tempted to live for today and ignore his needs in 30 or more years' time. Government protects him from this lack of foresight by ensuring health care and pensions for the old through direct supply and compulsory insurance.

Redistribution

The redistributive case for public intervention in the affairs of individuals is found across the whole spectrum of health and social policy. It is particularly associated with health, however, because of the tendency of politicians and philanthropists to view health as a fundamental element of life and a basic human right. More generally, however, an element of paternalism is also present. The poor may be given services rather than cash as a means of ensuring that they actually consume the service and do not spend the equivalent in money on activities frowned on by taxpaying donors. In Britain the redistributive argument is central to the foundations of the NHS but other countries, with no less claim to the ethics of redistribution, have chosen to redistribute health services by giving the poor the means to afford them rather than by supplying them directly to all without charge. Nonetheless, the NHS does have certain advantages, best seen perhaps by a wider consideration of the 'natural monopoly case'.

Monopoly

The basic objection to any monopoly is that it can exercise control over individuals in order to generate profits in excess of the cost of producing the commodity. The Organisation of Petroleum Exporting Countries (OPEC) has the power to generate millions of dollars of revenue and even to disrupt entire national economies by its price-fixing decisions. A natural monopoly is one where a single source of supply of a commodity is potentially the cheapest method of meeting the demand, that is, where a monopoly supplier is 'naturally' the most efficient. The obvious examples are services where the cost of installation is very high but after installation the cost of supplying an individual is relatively small. Railways, water and power supplies all have these characteristics. To have truly competing systems would require the duplication of extensive networks of rails, pipes or cables. Without this duplication, the consumer has little real choice of supplier, but the cost of duplication will be high because of the initial investment in building the second system. This cost will be spread over fewer users, and so the cost of the competing facilities will be higher for each of the competing suppliers than it would be for a single supplier. Yet without competition the consumer has no choice when faced with exorbitant prices charged by an unscrupulous monopolist.

The obvious natural monopoly with implications for health is the supply of water. Governments exercise controls over the quality of water supplied and also its cost. Any attempt by a water supplier to extract a very high price from consumers might damage health by reducing the amount used for effluent disposal. In addition, a high price for water, an essential for the maintenance of life, has implications for the ability of the poor to afford a healthy diet. Other monopolies, such as the supply of energy to households, are controlled by governments to prevent exploitation of consumers. But the health of consumers has also been used recently to justify intervention in the sale of gas and electricity. The high cost of energy in the late 1970s has led to growing concern that poor consumers may not consume enough to keep warm in winter. Hence, schemes to assist with the payment of energy costs have been introduced partly as a public health measure.

The hospital as a monopoly

Natural monopolies also exist in the supply of specific health services, such as hospitals. The rapid rise in the use of expensive technological equipment to augment medical and other hospital staff has led the general hospital to become an item requiring major capital expenditure in developed countries. Recent figures for the UK suggest that the capital cost of an acute hospital bed with the necessary supporting services is of the order of many thousands of pounds. Once a town has one hospital, all its care is in the hands of a single organisation. Competition requires the construction of a second hospital which brings choice at the expense of a higher set of costs all round as both the old and the new hospital attempt to recoup the capital cost from their share of patients. In the US recently the federal government has been trying to restrain the cost explosion in health services by limiting the number of facilities that are constructed to some norm based on the need for the service. However, this goes against traditional American policy towards the encouragement of competition and has recently been challenged in the courts by a hospital company seeking to compete in a town already well provided with beds.

To summarise, the essential feature of the natural monopoly is that a single source of supply is the cheapest method of meeting the local demand for the service or commodity, as long as the monopolist is prevented from extortionate pricing. Its efficiency rests on the high cost of building a competing facility. Government intervention acts as a substitute for competition to ensure that the price and quality of the service are acceptable.

The monopoly of medical knowledge

Aside from the expensive surroundings in which it is practised, medicine has a further monopoly characteristic. Medical knowledge is itself a monopoly, built up by a long and expensive period of investment in the training of the doctor. As the doctor has the monopoly on knowledge, he or she may take most of the decisions concerning the amount of health services that the consumer receives. To provide effective competition and prevent monopoly abuse would require a much larger supply of doctors so that every patient could obtain second and third opinions routinely but, yet again, this would increase the cost of investment in medical education. The absence of a second opinion leaves the patient potentially vulnerable to exploitation by quacks. Strict professional standards of education and ethics have been introduced to outlaw quackery and to prevent the exploitation of the patient. Many observers have argued that, given these safeguards, allowing the consumer some freedom to choose his doctor and his treatment is desirable for a number of reasons. Firstly, anything which encourages freedom of action encourages the transmission of demand from consumers to suppliers. In a planned economy, no matter how many people may desire high fashion shoes, for example, the central planners may decide nonetheless to invest in steel-making rather than shoe-making. In a market economy, if enough people want the shoes, someone somewhere will manufacture or import them. The wishes of the people are thus expressed rather than being suppressed by government. Thus, it is argued that freedom of choice helps to achieve expenditure on the things that people want rather than those that politicians want. The choice provides a form of decentralised democracy which allows people to pursue the things they want most. Secondly, freedom of choice gives the individual a greater awareness of a transaction. As a taxpayer, the individual is largely divorced from decisions about the supply of public health services whereas he is crucially involved if he pays the bill for his own care. It is argued that free provision from taxes encourages a kind of schizophrenia in which the individual demands a better service when acting as a consumer but is reluctant to pay in his role as taxpayer.

Demand for health care: leader or follower

Certainly, the argument above has much to recommend it for many commodities. People have different preferences for food and even the most socialist of governments has not enforced a standard pattern of food consumption. Freedom of choice allows minority tastes to be catered for and informs suppliers of changes in public attitudes. However, the argument cannot be transferred uncritically to the health service field. The whole concept of freedom of choice is undermined in medicine because the patient has little if any idea about the treatment he needs or the likely outcome. Demands for a treatment can no longer stem from the kind of experimentation with alternatives that is a part of the determination of tastes for food and drink. Rather, they will depend on the advice of the doctor together with fashion and whatever the patient thinks he knows about the treatment. An American woman's preference for a hysterectomy, an operation performed much more frequently in the USA than in the UK, may be argued to be worth meeting if it relieves her psychological stress, even in the absence of any overt symptoms (Pauly, 1979). A more extreme operation, preventive mastectomy, which is becoming quite frequent in the USA may also be defended as offering relief from the fear of cancer. However, this argument begs important questions about the way in which the demand is generated. If a woman finds herself in the minority of her age group who still have a womb, she may understandably feel a degree of unease. Peer pressure may generate the fear of disease which in turn generates the demand for treatment. In consequence, there may be a sense in which the demand for the hysterectomy is invalid in that it does not arise from the individual but is a consequence of the actions of others. Instead of freedom of choice, the individual is being led by the system towards the operation.

This kind of leading of demand takes place in all markets to a degree. Men and women are not born with every taste and preference inscribed on tablets of stone. Indeed, the first steps in the consumption of two commodities, alcohol and tobacco, are often associated with considerable distaste. The pressure to emulate contemporaries is usually enough to encourage the individual to overcome the initial repugnance and develop a taste for one or both commodities. However the individual's general inability to choose his medical care rationally and the lack of opportunities for learning by experience separate medicine from everyday consumption.

A further characteristic of the demand also casts doubt on the appropriateness of a system of supply that encourages patients to exercise choice. This is the method of payment for the service. Because of the growth of technological medicine, a great deal of health care is now too expensive for an individual to be able to afford from his current financial reserves. In consequence, private and public insurance systems are widespread. These have the effect of reducing the amount paid by the patient for the benefit of the doctor's knowledge. This in turn increases the scope for potential exploitation by reducing the patient's resistance to it. Normally, a customer will resist overcharging by a supplier if only because he ultimately runs out of money as the price escalates. However, if the cost of the service is being paid by someone else, he has no real stake in the financial side of the transaction and so has no incentive to resist the rising costs. Many observers have argued that the role of public and private insurance as the paymasters of American medicine has led to the rapid inflation in expenditure and services in the US health sector (e.g. Fuchs, 1974; Evans, 1974). Routine surgery for example takes place at rates two or three times higher than for similar populations in other developed countries. The doctor who prescribes surgery will usually have a financial interest in the operation taking place. The patient will usually be covered by his insurance for routine surgery and so has no financial interest in the operation. Indeed, for an operation such as hysterectomy, a patient aware that others have received the operation at the expense of her insurance company may feel that this is an opportunity to get something back in return for all the premiums paid.

However, we must be cautious in concluding that higher surgery rates in the US are purely the result of economic arrangements in the supply of care. As in epidemiology, great care must be taken when attempting to infer causation from observations. Faced with a particular patient, the ethical and the greedy doctor may both prescribe the same course of treatment; the former because he feels he is morally bound to do his utmost for his patient, the latter because he gets paid for the treatments that he gives.

In developed countries, the British NHS is at one extreme of a spectrum of methods of supply and payment for health services. Most of Europe operates a mixture of public and private insurance with a compulsory minimum cover in many countries. Doctors are frequently paid according to the service they provide and so have an incentive to provide more services than in the UK. In the US, a development alongside private practice is the Health Maintenance Organisation (HMO). Under this regime, doctors do not receive a fee for each item of service provided to patients. Rather, each HMO is a primary and acute health care service providing members with the service they need, with need assessed by the HMO's doctors. Members pay subscriptions to the HMO instead of purchasing private health insurance. Clearly, we might expect to find lower rates of operations in HMO's than in orthodox private practice. However, since the HMO is competing with private practice, it may have to appear to be doing as much for its members as private practice in order to retain them. Thus, it faces pressures towards providing more services even though in the short term it saves money if it provides less. The final test of HMO's will be their long-term effect on health and the cost of achieving it relative to private practice. However, an evaluation of this kind would require a great deal of detailed evidence and no definitive verdict can be determined as yet.

Public intervention: a summary

Public intervention in the health care field stems from at least four motives: to protect individuals from health risks or health care cost burdens generated by the behaviour of others; to protect them from themselves; to provide adequate health care for the poor; to protect individuals from the natural monopolies in the health care sector. These concerns have led governments throughout the developed world to legislate against certain activities and to subsidise the provision of health care, for some groups at least. In most developed countries, where physicians and other providers are paid according to the level of service given, public intervention in the health care market has not stemmed the tide of inflation in medical expenditure, and has frequently swelled it. The British NHS has been very successful in controlling the total budget. Proponents of this approach argue that it ensures that services are given to those in the greatest need. Critics argue that reliance on taxes inhibits the growth of the health care sector in response to genuine demand. In order to resolve the argument, a complex assessment of inputs and outcomes would be required. Without this, the reader should look with care at crude comparisons of expenditures. What is important is not how much each country spends on health services but the resources it can buy with that expenditure. Doubling the pay of the workers in the NHS tomorrow would not increase inputs or health even though it would raise expenditure to the level of other developed countries.

THE CHOICE OF OPTIONS

The economic arithmetic—benefits minus costs

A wholly rational choice between alternative methods of improving health with limited resources requires a detailed appraisal of costs and benefits. Chapter 5 has outlined the steps and pitfalls on the path to a rigorous epidemiological assessment of a single treatment. Choosing between alternative and widely differing options for the use of resources requires some comparison of different outcomes but this may be very difficult. Suppose for example, that three programmes are possible, any one of which will use up the total available budget. Programme A will extend the lives of those affected by more life years than B, and B by more than C. At first glance the choice is obvious. But what if A extends the lives of a group of 80 year-old patients by 1 year each while B and C offer appreciable gains in life expectancy to smaller numbers of younger people? Does the age of the beneficiaries lead us to change our initial view? Further complications arise if B leads to survival but with sustained physical impairment while C maintains full physical functioning of its smaller groups of beneficiaries. Age, disability, psychological state and other dimensions of the population groups that benefit may each lead us to modify the initial assessment based only on life years.

The comparison of different types of health improvement can be based on value judgements, that is, judgements of the value of alternatives which stem from ethical positions or beliefs. For example, a value judgement that medicine should seek to save every possible life, regardless of the length of likely survival or its quality, would have implications for the choice between heroic interventions and other medical options. The difficulty faced by a researcher seeking to identify the value placed on a health outcome is considerable. Typically, commodities and services are valued by markets, but many people would find this a repugnant basis for valuing the health of men and women. But if the market is not used as a reflection of the value judgements of many individuals then alternative methods must be used. Either mechanisms must be devised to identify collective values outside the market or some set of values must be imposed, perhaps at the whim of the decision maker. We may not like the implications of any of these methods of valuing health but a relative valuation is an essential implicit or explicit component of a non-random choice of options. Even a decision to use only one standard of health, e.g. life years, requires the value judgement that an extension of life for the dying is everywhere and always of more value than health improvements for the living. However, value judgements of this kind rest on personal ethical positions the philosophical underpinnings of which are not amenable to a simple analysis here. Therefore, the ethics of health assessment are not examined in detail in this chapter. Ideally, a public health programme should be chosen in the light of the values attached to its benefits by the public at large. In practice, this is unlikely to be feasible. Nonetheless, public health options can still be analysed in a number of ways. Firstly, outcomes can be ignored and attention focused only on the cost of each programme. Secondly, more detailed comparisons can be made of programmes explicitly assumed to offer the same outcome. Thirdly, attempts can be made to assess outcomes in full, using a variety of value judgements to identify those which most influence the decision and so require endorsement or rejection by public decision-makers.

The cost of the option

We have already noted that limited budgets prevent society from pursuing every possible health programme at once. Money is the usual yardstick but budgets may be specified in manpower or other terms. In practice, the budget may depend on the choice to be made. The choice of cases for an operating theatre session, for example, will depend on the staff and time budgets available to a surgical firm in the NHS rather than on a cash budget. In such a choice, the input costs of alternatives to the consultant are the staff and time used by each case. Thus, costs should be viewed as wider than simply money, though money may frequently offer advantages as a measure which can be applied to a wide range of different inputs.

An informed choice can begin only when the costs, broadly defined, of each alternative are known. Benefits may remain vague but cost data at least ensure that appropriate comparisons are made. For example, it would be obviously unreasonable to reject a scheme offering little improvement without regard to the cost, high or low, of achieving it. Once the input required for each option is known, a choice which reconciles the cost in total inputs with the budget available can be made. A simple cost analysis of the kind above is undertaken frequently in the NHS when authorities draw up plans for the development of separate parts of the service and vote on a final plan.

What is the cost?

However, costing must be approached with caution. The costs of interest in an economic appraisal are the marginal opportunity costs. The marginal cost is the change in costs that occurs specifically because of the change in activities that is being considered. The opportunity cost is the loss of other useful opportunities which follows from the use of resources to provide the new activity. Both concepts are probably most easily seen in an example. Suppose an additional health service is to be provided. If it requires the provision of a building, the hiring of staff and the purchase of equipment and the materials then all of these will be marginal costs. The use of each type of resource will mean the loss of an opportunity to use it in some other way. For example, the use of silver to make an X-ray film means there is a little less silver available for ornaments or jewellery. The loss of the alternative use will be reflected by its price. Similarly, if staff employed by the health service are drawn away from other types of employment then the opportunity cost of using them in the health service is the output lost in the other job. This will be reflected by the wage rate paid in the job, a wage the health service must meet to recruit labour. Thus, the wage indicates the opportunity cost of labour.

It may frequently be the case that the true marginal cost of a service is quite different from the average cost estimates that are readily calculable. For example, hospitals frequently have empty rooms which must be heated to prevent maintenance problems. Therefore, if such a room is used to house an X-ray machine, no building or heating costs would be incurred. Projections of the cost per square foot for the room and the cost of heating based on averages for the whole hospital building would be misleading as the bills for the building and heating would be unaffected by the new service.

Alternatively, the new service may simply require the use of an existing machine that is not used throughout the day. In this case, the marginal cost of the additional X-ray service may be only the film, the electricity used to take the picture and perhaps some developing fluid. If the work can be accommodated within the department without any additional staffing then there is no marginal labour cost from the service. A higher rate of use may lead to more frequent maintenance of the machine or its more rapid deterioration and replacement. In this event, the relevant costs are the changes in the amount and timing of expenditure on new equipment. Alternatively, staff may be required to work overtime at above average rates of pay in order to accommodate the extra work. In this case, the marginal cost will be the change in the department wage bill following the introduction of the new service.

To summarise, the marginal opportunity cost of a change in the services provided is measured in terms of the actual changes in the total cost of the staff and other resources used to provide the service. Where a new service can be accommodated with little change, the marginal cost will be low and the service will be worth providing even if the expected outcome is small. Conversely, where the service requires the additional purchase of buildings and all inputs to the process including staff, the marginal cost will be high and will only be justified by a higher expected outcome. Before we go on to examine the difficulties of assessing the outcomes of health services for an economic appraisal, it is important to note one final aspect of costing in the health services.

Costing hospitals

Hospitals are characterised by the very high proportion of their total expenditure devoted to the employment of staff. Of the order of 70 per cent of a UK hospital's costs are made up of wages and salaries. The important difference between men and machines in any job is that manpower can be used flexibly to perform a variety of tasks or to vary the time spent on each task whereas a machine will be rigidly constructed to complete specific tasks at a specific pace. Medical and nursing staff devote their time to a wide variety of cases. If necessary, they may be able to cope with a heavier workload from time to time. As long as they do cope, no extra (i.e. marginal) cost appears in the hospital wage bill. The real cost imposed by extra work is the foregone opportunity to spend more time on another of their tasks. As the workload rises and the amount of time given to each patient falls, the quality of care may deteriorate. This may be because the faster pace of activity increases the risk of error, because the need to hurry reduces the extent to which each task is completed or because important communication with the patient is foregone.

As long as the particular task to be costed occupies only a small part of the working time of a member of staff (such as the care of one patient with a particular diagnosis in a ward of 30 or the care of one diagnostic group in a specialty treating 20 or 30 different disorders) separate costing of the activity will be difficult. For example, domiciliary care may be better in medical or social terms for a particular group of patients. However, keeping that group out of hospital will save no money on the hospital wage bill unless the group is large enough to permit the closure of a ward or the reduction of staff. The need for accurate analysis usually limits epidemiological studies to comparatively narrow ranges of conditions, each of which may be too small to have an impact on the hospital's costs when domiciliary care is introduced. If the required domiciliary services can be provided by the hospital staff making home visits then the preferred option of home care may be readily implemented. However, if this is impossible, extra expenditure may be required. Although domiciliary care may use less staff time than hospital care, if staff time cannot be redeployed to the community then no savings occur in hospital to offset the expenditure on domiciliary care.

When looking at costs, the relevant cost is the marginal opportunity cost, the sacrifices that must be made if the new activity is to be undertaken. Costing is at its simplest when the unit size of the inputs affected by the decision is close in size to the units in which the change is to be measured. For example, one extra X-ray requires one extra film, but less than 1 per cent of the time of a radiographer and radiologist. The film is readily costed, the staff are not. Readers should particularly be aware of the misleading use of average costs instead of marginal costs. Many a project has been undertaken in the health field on the expectation that estimated savings (wrongly based on average costs) would offset the cost of the new development.

The costs to others

The obvious outcome of any programme in community medicine is health improvement. However, before examining the ways in which health improvements are dealt with, it is important not to overlook another aspect of outcome, costs that fall outside the original budget. Suppose, for example, that a health authority is examining options for home and hospital care for a disease. Within its own expenditure budget, it may be possible to provide more home care. But a consequence of a decision to reduce hospital care may be the imposition of costs on patients' families. Spouses or children may be required to give up their time, possibly their jobs, in order to provide home care. Although this costs the health authority nothing, it has a cost nonetheless.

We have already used the broad definition of cost adopted by economists, equating a cost with any loss of a useful commodity or opportunity. If a relative gives up work, society loses his production. If he gives up leisure, he has lost the opportunity to relax, which obviously is of value to him. A broad definition of cost is necessary to prevent mistaken decisions. A decision to 'save' by cutting health services is less of a saving for the taxpayer if he is obliged to accept other restrictions on his activity to care for his relatives. The lost recreation might be valued more highly than the tax cut he receives.

In an ideal analysis, the costs that are generated outside the initial budget, together with the benefits of the programme, will be included in the assessment. In practice, these costs are frequently difficult to assess, for example if relatives prefer to look after the patient or if they find his presence at home less worrying than hospitalisation, but they should not be overlooked, particularly in more straightforward cases where costs are generated for other agencies. Society as a whole may take the wrong decisions if health and local authorities each look only at the costs on their own budgets and ignore the effects of decisions on each other.

Outcomes—the cost-effective means to a given end

The identification of the various benefits from a health programme is the concern of the epidemiologist. Much of the earlier discussion in this book has focused on the methods used and the results obtained. Making these health benefits commensurate with money costs is a highly controversial method of analysis for choosing between options. Before examining the particular problems of valuation in money terms, we will look at a less problematic approach, cost-effectiveness analysis.

Cost-effectiveness analysis provides a method of choosing between alternatives that generate the same health benefits using different inputs at different costs. If the least cost method is chosen, then the largest number of patients can be treated from the available budget.

A recent example of the approach compared methods of delivering oxygen to patients with chronic respiratory problems who need to breathe extra oxygen for a large part of the day (Lowson et al, 1981). The alternatives were routine delivery of gas or liquid to the patients' homes or the installation of equipment which extracts oxygen directly from the air. Either way, the patient receives the necessary supply of oxygen and so the benefit of the service will be the same under each regime. Thus, the problems of assessing benefit itself are avoided. Given a commitment to support this group of patients, at the expense of treating some other care group, the choice of method can be made solely in terms of the costs.

Simple cost-effectiveness analysis, using a common unit of health benefit to compare programmes and policies, is a useful method of evaluating alternative options. It can highlight contradictions in existing policy by showing discrepancies in the amount spent to achieve a particular result by different means. For example, governments legislate on a wide range of matters in order to prevent premature death and the implied value of life inherent in each policy can be calculated approximately. Mooney (1977) shows that building standards, legislated after the collapse of the Ronan Point flats, imply a value of life as high as £20 million whereas child-proof drug containers were not introduced by legislation even though it is estimated that the cost per life saved would have been as low as £2000. Both estimates may be subject to some error, because of the difficulties of calculating exactly the lives saved by each measure. However, the order of magnitude of the difference is so great as to call into question the decisions to accept the first policy and reject the second.

One major complication which undermines cost-effectiveness analysis is the difficulty of ensuring that treatments compared have the same effects on physical and social functioning. The complexity of the human body is such that identical outcomes from different treatments cannot be predicted with any certainty and the evaluation may be obliged to await the results of long term follow-up of patients. A cost-effectiveness study of injection-compression treatment and surgical stripping for varicose veins (Piachaud & Weddell, 1972) found that the former was the lower cost method of relieving the problem. However, the 5 year follow-up of patients found that the relapse rate was much higher in the injection-compression treatment group (Beresford et al, 1978). Thus it could no longer be viewed as equally effective. One solution would be to alter the outcome measure from the idea of a cure to that of years of relief from symptoms. It might be cost-effective to give an inferior treatment to 5 patients, relieving their symptoms for 4 years on average, rather than to treat 1 patient by the best and most expensive method in order to give him 10 years relief. Indeed, it is worth emphasising the implication of the typical medical concern to give the best possible treatment to a patient. The best for one may mean nothing at all for other patients or potential patients. Even the crudest comparative appraisal of treatments should not lose sight of this.

Valuing the outcome—cost-benefit analysis

The weakness of cost-effectiveness analysis is that it can only be used to compare options offering a similar—ideally an identical—outcome. The evaluation of alternative methods of supplying oxygen to chronic respiratory cases tells us nothing about the general desirability of doing this at all compared to some other use of public funds. Life-years gained or time free from pain offer a common yardstick by which diverse health options can be compared and such comparisons could be extended further if a widely accepted and easily assessed health index could be derived for patients of all types. Points on the health index would then become the common outcome of all options and the cost-effective choices made. The complexity of health, affecting all the subtle dimensions of human life, make such an indicator somewhat utopian. Nonetheless, a number of attempts have been made to extend the evaluation by attaching a monetary value to the health outcomes. This widens the comparative framework so that health options can be compared with those in fields such as transport or energy supply. The methods involved are termed cost-benefit analysis.

Clearly, every rational decision between alternative courses of action must rest on some assessment of the advantages and disadvantages, the costs and benefits, of each. However, cost benefit analysis is usually defined more specifically to cover appraisals where the benefits are calculated in monetary terms so as to be directly comparable with the costs. Much of the detailed research of this kind in the UK has been focused on the transport sector. Transport development has implications for the time spent travelling and the congestion of alternative means of travel. Not all the benefits of these two aspects may be captured by the projected price of the new service. For example, if one individual uses the railway instead of his car, all road users receive a slight benefit. Cheaper fares might encourage more rail travel and make the reduction in congestion appreciable yet the road users who benefit face no direct charge for the rail service which gives them a benefit. Similarly, an airport close to a major conurbation will save air travellers some time. Half an hour saved may not provoke a rush to cross the Atlantic but may nonetheless be of value. The difficulty in transport appraisals lies in the choice of an appropriate wage or price for time saved by motorists or air travellers. One solution is to use the going wage rate for the people involved, but this overlooks the way in which the time is actually used. A saving of time on a journey may be dissipated in a range of activities, each of which is done slightly more slowly. The benefits of a few extra minutes in the bath or the second cup of coffee at breakfast may not be valued very highly. In consequence, it is usual to find a range of prices used in cost-benefit analysis to identify the point at which a particular price becomes critical to the acceptance or rejection of the option on the basis of its costs and benefits. For example, the decision on the location of an airport may hinge on an environmental impact. The final political decision on a site will then imply a particular price for the environmental effects. Consistency would suggest that other projects with an environmental effect should be similarly treated.

In practice, cost-benefit analysis has a chequered history. The mass of detail involved in an appraisal of a project such as the Third London Airport is such that no single value can be extracted as the pivot on which the decision turns. It is therefore no surprise to find that the end of that appraisal was political rejection of the apparently most beneficial site followed by shelving of the whole programme.

Valuing life

Any evaluation of health improvements in money terms is more complex and more emotive than similar appraisal of transport. For example, the approach has been used in an attempt to demonstrate the benefits of heart transplantation over the costs in money terms (Haberman, 1980). The analysis rests on the valuation of a return to work by the patient in terms of his wages, social security and taxes.

The weakness of the productive labour approach is that the value of life will depend on the personal characteristics of the individual and his net contribution to the rest of society. In such a crude calculus the old and unemployed would be valued below others. Haberman's study has several weaknesses but the approach, if appropriately conducted, does provide a minimum measure of benefit. If we accept that life has an intrinsic value over and above the value of one individual's contribution in work, then the benefits from saving life would exceed the purely productive benefits. This in turn means that programmes which yield benefits, calculated from earnings, which exceed the costs of achieving them are highly beneficial and even programmes which do not have production benefits that offset costs may be beneficial because of the intrinsic value of the life saved.

The reader who finds the whole question of placing a money value on life repugnant should not overlook the fact that every decision to use manpower and resources to produce something other than a life-saving commodity or service has implicit in it a value of life. It is not the economist who is responsible for the scarcity of resources which prevent every desirable commodity being obtained. Rather, he seeks to clarify the choices and increase the consistency with which they are made.

Consistency requires that the benefits of the widest range of alternatives be evaluated before a decision is made. This is easily seen in the case of heart transplants. Putting aside possible technical reservations, Haberman has apparently shown that the benefits of heart transplantation exceed the costs: but this need not signal the expansion of the transplant programme. There may be many other uses of the resources which would yield greater benefits still. Given an appraisal of all programmes, we can then rank them in terms of the benefits expected to accrue. We might then find that heart transplantation is no longer an attractive investment, for two reasons. Firstly, many treatments or preventive measures may be more beneficial for the same cost, pushing transplants further down the list of priorities. Secondly, we might find a growing reluctance on the part of the public to bear the cost of a health sector big enough to accommodate all the beneficial programmes. As each programme is adopted in turn, the resources available to meet other desires will dwindle. The decline in living standards implied will almost certainly be accompanied by a growing reluctance to fund yet more health services. That is, the opportunity cost of foregoing a further pound's worth of consumption will be higher because people value that pound's worth more as living standards fall. For example, a man who dines out every evening may regard the foregoing of one such meal a month as a small price to pay for a life-saving health programme, even one with quite limited benefit. However, when the health sector has grown, and reduced his consumption of restaurant meals to one per month, he may be less ready to sacrifice a further dinner per month for another health programme. Essentially, the individual and society as a whole are faced with the choice between more of life and a higher standard of the living of it. Since people frequently engage in activities which damage their health, in full knowledge of the risks involved, it is doubtful if the choice of expenditure options would be that which maximised expenditure on health improving programmes.

The evaluation in money terms of life itself or of other dimensions of health remains a comparative rarity in cost-benefit studies. Most economists would argue that a cost-benefit exercise is more appropriately seen as a way of structuring the evaluation of options rather than as the mechanism for choosing a preferred option. The advantages of the method are that it requires resource costs to be specified in detail and that it makes explicit relevant benefits which are frequently treated in only vague terms. Epidemiology has contributed a great deal to the identification of benefits from treatment. The economic approach can then be viewed as a step towards the resolution of choice between alternative programmes of demonstrable health benefit. However, the final step in the choice decision will invariably be political, involving the value judgements of legislative or executive bodies prepared for reasons of political benefit to commit the necessary resources to the option selected. Anything which helps to illuminate these value judgements may help to ensure that the choices made are consistently in the best interests of the community and not merely in the best interests of those making the decision.

Economic choices

To conclude, the essence of the economic approach is that benefits are only achievable at the expense of alternative benefits. Failure to perceive the opportunity costs of achieving a health improvement will lead to inappropriate choices being made. For example, the total elimination of all man-made air pollution is a laudable sentiment. However, to turn this sentiment into a policy is to ignore the cost of its achievement. In the early 1950s, smog was established as a major cause of respiratory disease and mortality. Its removal from big cities in the UK through legislation on smoke emission was not costless but it was facilitated by the widespread availability of coke, a smokeless fuel by-product of the production of town gas. Thus, the cost impact of the enforced change in fuel was reduced. The present levels of air pollution in the UK arise principally from industrial processes, and from road transport. Pollution can be reduced from both these sources and much of it is already removed from the first. However, the cost of eliminating industrial pollution cannot be ignored. The marginal cost of successive reductions in the level of pollution is likely to rise as the pollution level falls. It may be easy to filter emissions from a chimney but much more difficult to prevent fugitive emissions of dust from the general area of the process. Where the pollution is already scattered in this way, the cost of filtering may be small compared to the cost of gathering the affected air so that filtering can take place. The desirability of incurring such costs will depend crucially on the anticipated benefits. For a product such as asbestos, which can be highly damaging to the human lung even at low concentrations, a very high cost might be regarded as worth paying to prevent loss of life and respiratory disease. For other kinds of industrial pollution, the gains from reductions from already low levels of pollution to zero are equivocal. The cost in terms of lost jobs or exports may be appreciable if pollution reduction is costly. For road transport, the health hazards of pollution have recently undergone renewed scrutiny and it is argued by some that important health improvements could be achieved by a reduction in the lead content of petrol. The gains are for the epidemiologist to assess. Estimates of the cost effect of lead removal vary but in terms of the price per gallon of petrol, most appear small compared to the annual price rises inflicted by the Exchequer. Thus it may be perfectly consistent to seek elimination of one form of pollution but not of another, from their present levels, because of the different marginal costs of each programme.

To sum up, the economic approach to the appraisal of health or any other set of alternative programmes is to pose two questions.

1. What must we give up for this programme?
2. How do the programme benefits compare with those given up?

Obliging the proponents of any health option to answer these two questions to the fullest extent possible is the only basis for a consistent health policy. Mistakes will still occur, if only because of the difficulty and time required to obtain a complete picture of health outcomes. However, the routine asking of these questions would leave the satisfaction that only with hindsight could things have been done better.

REFERENCES

Atkinson A B, Meade T W 1974 Methods and preliminary findings in assessing the economic and health service consequences of smoking with particular reference to lung cancer. Journal of the Royal Statistical Society. Series A 137 3: 333–46

Atkinson A B, Townsend J 1977 Economic aspects of reduced smoking. Lancet: 492–4

Beresford S A A, Chant A D B, Jones H O, Piachaud D, Weddell J M 1978 Varicose veins: a comparison of surgery and injection compression sclerotherapy—a five year follow-up. Lancet 1: 921–4

Evans R G 1974 Supplier-induced demand: some empirical evidence, and implications. In: Perlman M (ed) The economics of health and medical care. Macmillan Press, London

Fuchs V R 1974 Who shall live? Health economics and social choice. Basic Books, New York

Haberman S 1980 Putting a price on life. Health and Social Science Journal, 4th July

Lowson K V, Drummond M F, Bishop J M 1981 Costing new services: long-term domiciliary oxygen therapy. Lancet I: 1146

Mooney G H 1977 The valuation of life. Macmillan, London

Pauly M V 1979 What is unnecessary surgery? Milbank Memorial Fund Quarterly; Health and Society 57: 1, 95–117

Piachaud D, Weddell J M 1972 The cost of treating varicose veins Lancet 2: 1191–2

FURTHER READING

Culyer A J 1976 Need and the National Health Service. Martin Robertson, London
This book, written for non-specialists, gives an economist's perspective on the

problems of meeting competing health service demands with limited budgets. As well as dealing lucidly with some of the conceptual questions it focuses on a range of practical problems.

Drummond M F 1980 Principles of economic appraisal in health: an introduction. Martin Robertson, London
Again for a non-technical audience, this book explains the principles of cost-effectiveness and cost-benefit appraisal of health programmes.

Cullis J G, West P A 1979 The economics of health: an introduction. Martin Robertson, London
Although in parts accessible to the non-specialist, this book is primarily for those who have mastered some basic economic theory, though the volumes above would provide an alternative grounding. It is a text-book treatment of the theory and application of economics in the health field.

7

From policy formation to health service management

In the previous chapter the grounds for public intervention were laid out. This chapter continues this theme and examines the practical constraints upon intervention and the alternative forms that intervention has taken in the provision of health-related services in the British context.

Under the National Health Service Acts of 1946 and 1977 duties are laid upon the Secretary of State to promote a comprehensive health service designed to secure improvement in (1) the physical and mental health of the people and (2) the prevention, diagnosis and treatment of illness. The word comprehensive was intended to have two interpretations, ensuring coverage of all people living in the UK and covering all necessary forms of treatment. Within these very broad aims the NHS has no publicly declared objectives to be met by its services. As a consequence the NHS is based on policies or priorities which change with events and governments (HMSO, 1979). Decisions to proceed in one direction or another tend therefore to be pragmatic responses to current circumstances rather than the product of detailed planning.

Policies often take the form of broad guidelines for action which the Government chooses to promote and there are a number of ways in which the Government may exert its influence. The choice of method is determined by what can be described as an unwritten constitution relating to health matters. This chapter examines various approaches taken by British governments and outlines the main features of this unwritten constitution which limits the extent of government intervention.

PRESSURES TO CREATE POLICY

It is rarely clear why particular issues become a legitimate concern of policy makers, although there are a number of ways in which their attention might be gained. These issues may be highlighted by research findings: by concern from within a government or health service department about the efficiency and effectiveness of some of its policies; the mass media may decide to promote an issue; a pressure group may mount a campaign to attract public and political attention; questions may be asked in Parliament or within a local policy making body. Often policies seem to be the result of a culmination of pressure from some or all of these sources, in many cases over a period of years.

For example the recent trend towards moving long stay patients from hospital to community care has a variety of origins. Evidence for the benefits to be derived from moving people from institutional care to care in their own homes can be traced back to the nineteenth century. Care at home for the sick and elderly who could be suitably looked after by their own families was considered by some authorities to be a cheaper and more humanitarian alternative to the punitive atmosphere of the workhouse. During the early years of the twentieth century the idea of home care as a substitute for institutional care was lost as it became common for only highly dependent patients and children to be housed in institutions. In 1913 the Mental Deficiency Act allowed voluntary and statutary authorities to make provisions for the mentally handicapped in the community. The 1946 NHS Act extended these arrangements for the care and aftercare of illness and mental defectiveness. The emphasis here had shifted from care by institutions to care provided by local authority services.

The first real drive against institutional care came with a speech made by Enoch Powell in 1961 in which he announced his intentions to halve the number of hospital beds for mental patients over the following 14 years. Justification for this stemmed from belief in the effectiveness of the new psychotropic drugs introduced in the 1950's even though there was no evidence to suggest whether these contributed to recovery or merely alleviated symptoms.

In the 1960s the emphasis on the community was extended to encompass geriatric patients, the mentally ill, the physically and mentally handicapped and women in childbirth. This intention was documented in two publications, 'A hospital plan' (HMSO, 1962) and 'Health and welfare: the development of community care' (HMSO, 1963), which recommended increasing local authority responsibility for those client groups. The major impetus for the move from hospital to the community came from the belief that it was cheaper to help people at home than in institutions. Besides, in the 1960s a series of sociological publications demonstrated that institutions had a damaging effect upon their inmates. Goffman's work on asylums became the basis for many arguments about such effects (Goffman, 1963).

Allegations made in a Sunday newspaper of ill treatment of patients in Ely hospital led to a government inquiry. The report published in 1969 supported the allegations. This, and further attacks by the mass media added fuel to the arguments in favour of removing people from institutions. However, during the 1970s few constructive ideas were put forward as to what should be done for people transferred to the community. Research concentrated on trying to determine ways in which voluntary and family support could be used to help care for people at home. Many organisations and self help groups were developed during this decade with central government support and financial aid. Joint consultative committees were introduced to facilitate cooperation between the health and local authority social services departments and policy innovations in this area were encouraged by providing central government funds to finance new schemes (for a more detailed account see Jones et al, 1978).

RESPONSIBILITY AND SOCIAL POLICY

A major facet of policy decisions is concerned with determining where the responsibility for policy implementation lies. Should this be the individual, the health professional, a local decision making body or the Government itself? The following examples highlight the different courses of action that have been pursued in the implementation of policy and the economic, ethical, political and circumstantial factors which have moulded the final decisions.

Individual responsibility

As more information relating to modifiable risk factors has become available, the Government has felt a duty to encourage a responsible attitude in society towards personal health. At all possible opportunities it seeks to promote this personal responsibility by encouraging approved 'healthy behaviours'. Consequently action has been taken to improve public knowledge of risks to health and to promote the transmission of information about such risks to members of the public. It has attempted this in a number of ways: firstly by publishing booklets on certain risks to health such as excess alcohol and poor diet; secondly, through the agency of the Health Education Council which promotes the benefits to be derived from healthy living; and thirdly by offering support and encouragement to the media who have tried to promote health education. The main emphasis of this approach has been limited to encouraging individual members of the public to take action on their own initiative to improve their health.

Any government must be certain that it is acting in the long term best interests of its people and that it is not offering ill considered advice which could damage both health and political credibility. In many cases the Government seeks advice from permanent bodies of experts called together to review current and past evidence and to advise on the best way of proceeding. The experts, in turn, may be influenced by the reports and thoughts of other bodies, professional and lay, which are similarly concerned about particular issues.

Throughout the 1950s and 1960s the scientific journals reported evidence on the possible relationships between nutrition and cardiovascular disease. Medical and public concern grew because some of the evidence indicated that there might be benefits from replacing saturated with polyunsaturated fats in the diet. Indeed, one polyunsaturated margarine manufacturer based its sales promotion campaign on the idea that its product would actually improve the health of those who ate it. Such claims had to be examined by the Food Standards Committee to ensure that the public was not being misled. In June 1970 the Committee on the Medical Aspects of Food Policy (COMA) set up a specialist panel to determine whether there was any evidence to substantiate the hypothesised relationship between nutrition and cardiovascular disease. The preface stated that the report 'represents a distillation by long and critical discussion of facts that might be relevant to the formulation of food policy in the United Kingdom' (DHSS, 1974). The panel's job was confined to an interpretation of the evidence concerning the influence, composition and amount of fat in the diet on the death rate from coronary heart disease. Their recommendations were cautious. Obesity should be avoided and saturated fat and sucrose intake should be reduced, but the Committee could not be certain that an intake of polyunsaturated fats would reduce the risk of heart disease.

In 1976 a joint working party of the Royal College of Physicians of London and the British Cardiac Society reported on the prevention of coronary heart disease (Journal of the Royal College of Physicians, 1976). They aimed to offer medical practitioners the best advice based on research up to that time. Less cautious than COMA, they recommended that for the whole community there should be a reduction in the amount of saturated fats. Other recommendations concerned the reduction of cigarette smoking, increased physical activity and the recording of blood pressures.

The Chief Medical Officer at the DHSS sent copies to all doctors drawing attention to the similarities and differences between this and the 1974 report. COMA then reconsidered its findings, in relation to the 1976 report and concluded that no new evidence had been provided which would substantiate the theory that a higher intake of polyunsaturates would reduce the death rate from heart disease. In fact some of the evidence seemed to demonstrate that high levels of polyunsaturated fats might be themselves harmful to health.

In 1975 the Social Services and Employment sub-committee of the House of Commons Expenditure Committee began a special enquiry into preventive medicine. The Expenditure Committee was concerned about the increasing cost of the NHS and also that a very high proportion of NHS resources was devoted solely to hospital service. The report (HMSO, 1977a) made 58 recommendations which covered the whole area of preventive medicine. Some of these concerned the diet of different groups in the population, and recommended that information about fats should be published to encourage people to moderate their fat intake or switch to polyunsaturated fats. The government accepted the first, but the second only with reservations. The acceptance of the recommendations was published in a White Paper presented to Parliament in December 1977.

The White Paper stated the position of the Government in relation to dietary policy. 'In connection with diet the role of Government is directed primarily towards assembling, assessing and disseminating information, based on scientific evidence on which individuals can base their own actions. Issues in this field are complex. Individuals' metabolism and material circumstances vary and the present relationship between diet and health is incomplete. It is far from easy for the Government to produce clear straightforward advice applicable to the public generally' (HMSO, 1977a). The White Paper recognised that it was often more appropriate to bring facts to the attention of those professionally concerned with diet and health and let them advise individuals.

In the absence of any further evidence since the 1974 report, the White Paper stated that the Government was unable to accept that polyunsaturated fats should be regarded as a simple alternative for saturated fats. The section on diet concluded by noting the importance of placing before the public up-to-date medical and scientific knowledge, but it was felt that nutritional considerations should only have an indirect effect on food policy. 'In the Government's view the total pattern of demand for food should represent the sum of informed choices freely made by the members of the public'. Thus this food policy has been restricted to minimal intervention in the lives of individuals and controls have been limited to informing individuals of the risks to their health rather than controlling the availability of the possibly harmful foods. This latter option is only used in cases where there is more than reasonable doubt about the harmful effects of certain foods or substances.

Service responsibility

Stemming directly from the need for individuals to minimise risks to their own health, the Government has also had to consider the benefits to be gained from the early diagnosis of disease through screening programmes. Screening is a process which attracts much public attention. The objective of identifying a disease before it becomes debilitating and at the point at which cure might be effective is appealing. The treatment services of the NHS place the responsibility for seeking medical care firmly upon the patient. With the exception of accidents and mental illness, the potential patient has to determine when to seek attention from his general practitioner who then assesses the patient's need for treatment at his own hands or refers him to the more expensive resources of the hospital and its specialist services.

This 'gatekeeping' procedure for determining need and thereby rationing limited health service resources is disturbed by the introduction of a screening programme. The responsibility for initiating contact with the health services is transferred from the patient to the service providers who have a duty to promote the welfare of patients. A characteristic of screening programmes is that they generate expectations and hence demand within the population at which they are directed over and above what the health service is geared up to provide and can afford within its limited budget. Where large increases in demand are expected it would be impossible for a health authority to finance screening programmes without additional central government monies. As a consequence, the initiation and promotion of national screening programmes are left to central policy until a programme becomes fully established when it can be delegated, as in the case of cervical screening, to a local level.

To ensure that a screening programme is scientifically, ethically, and economically acceptable it should conform to the basic criteria of Wilson and Jungner which are detailed in Chapter 4. Even though screening programmes may be justified according to these criteria, allocation of responsibility for carrying them out and the way in which they should be operated are matters of policy. Central government might institute a nationwide screening programme, or local health authorities could be called upon to create their own programmes. The degree to which service providers promote uptake of their services is also variable. Inviting members of the public to use screening facilities as and when they choose places less responsibility on the service providers than schemes which actively pursue people at work or in their own homes.

As screening techniques are developed, programmes become eligible for policy debate. Amniocentesis screening for spina bifida was known to be possible after the discovery that high concentrations of alphafetoprotein (AFP) in the amniotic fluid indicated the presence of anencephaly and open spina bifida. It was apparent that such a programme would be very expensive in terms of medical manpower. This, combined with the risks of spontaneous abortion due to amniocentesis, meant that policy makers were reluctant to support a national programme of routine screening for spina bifida. But when it was found that the presence of neural tube defects was associated with a raised level of AFP in maternal serum (detected by a relatively cheap and low risk technique) it became possible to think in terms of local programmes to determine which pregnant women were at risk. The more expensive and hazardous amniocentesis could then be performed on this restricted group.

One much discussed programme has been multiphasic screening which has achieved great popularity in France where it is offered as part of the occupational health schemes. The South East London Screening Study undertaken between 1967 and 1977 cast doubts on the usefulness of such programmes. The researchers concluded that none of the measures of outcome, mortality, morbidity or health service usage was improved by screening (South East London Screening Study Group, 1977). The failure to detect objective evidence of benefit from the screening justified the withholding of the vast outlay of resources required to mount a national programme. Multiphasic screening cannot yet be justified on scientific, ethical or economic grounds, and in consequence the British Government has not felt it possible to promote its introduction.

National responsibility

In some cases individuals cannot act to minimise risks to their health because these risks lie outside their personal control. In such instances the Government has accepted a duty to take action at a national level to minimise these risks to individual health. In many cases there are competing considerations to be taken into account. Punitive legislative measures are often unpopular with voters and powerful groups such as industries, and the long term economic consequences of some measures outweigh the direct benefits to individuals. The Government has preferred to invite voluntary cooperation from tobacco companies to work out ways of reducing the amount of tar in cigarettes and to limit the promotional activity undertaken. As Chapter 6 has already mentioned, cigarette taxes generate income for governments and also it is possible that smoking reduces the life expectancy of those who would otherwise be drawing retirement pensions for longer periods. Economic considerations are also likely to prevent extreme actions such as banning cigarettes. Such considerations have, however, also led to the introduction of policies which can improve health.

Malnutrition and health

At the turn of the century, there was concern that some children were too hungry or too ill to benefit from education services. As a consequence the 1906 Education (provision of meals) Act empowered local authorities to provide meals to children in need and legislation in 1907 started medical inspections of schoolchildren. Throughout the inter-war years both the Ministry of Health and the Board of Education continued to insist that the only purpose of school medical and dental services was to remove health defects which prevented children from learning.

In 1931 a committee of eminent nutritionists was set up to give expert advice on the effects of poverty on malnutrition. The first report was full of disagreements between members. The whole debate was confused by the inability of researchers to agree on precise definitions of malnutrition, poverty and health. The Ministry of Health was committed to denying any relationship between health and malnutrition. It argued that no accurate tests existed to substantiate the relationship. Other more general indicators such as mortality rates showed that the health of the population was constantly improving. In 1933 the British Medical Association committee on nutrition entered the debate and recommended a daily intake of 3400 calories per man, which it suggested was possible on the then current rates of unemployment benefit. The Ministry of Health reacted violently to the report and accused the committee of having no experts in nutrition and of discussing issues outside their remit such as the cost of food. The Ministry remained adamant that there was no evidence that malnutrition existed and even if it did it was not related to low income but to ignorance of how to prepare and cook food.

Throughout the 1930s the Government and the expert committees who advised it refused to recognise the relationship between health, nutrition and low income. This was presumably because to have done so would have required positive action which the depressed national economy could not afford.

Pressure groups sprang up to contest the Ministry's attitude: a group of doctors formed the Committee Against Malnutrition; the Trades Union Congress and the Labour Party announced their commitment to the association between malnutrition and poverty; an organisation called the Children's Minimum Council was created. These groups lobbyed Parliament with demands for daily rations of milk for all children at state-aided schools and free school milk for all needy children. In 1934 the Government did make it possible for schoolchildren to purchase one third of a pint of milk a day for one halfpenny though this would be free for the needy. Disappointingly this policy could not be attributed to the work of the malnutrition lobby. It was the National Milk Publicity Council, concerned about boosting milk consumption who persuaded the Government to introduce the school milk policy. (For a more detailed account see McNichol, 1980.)

It often appears that government health departments tend to take a back seat in government policy making. One explanation of this is that health departments do not generate income, they merely use national resources. Income generating departments such as defence and industry have more power to defend their interests, which are often concerned with promoting national, economic welfare rather than individual personal welfare. In general, where one Ministry determines that a certain policy might bring it into disrepute, the benefits for another less politically powerful Ministry are often disregarded. In 1978 the Minister of Transport announced that he would not make the wearing of seatbelts compulsory because he valued individual freedom. The money that could have been saved for the NHS by preventing traffic related injuries was disregarded because of other political interests. The legislation making the wearing of seatbelts compulsory was ultimately enacted as a result of a Private Member's Bill introduced by an individual Member of Parliament rather than as a result of ministerial initiative.

Air pollution

A similar story of political wrangling over health policies can be found in relation to air pollution. Some of the background to the study of air pollution is described in Chapter 3. The modern story begins following the London smog of 1952, in which many lives were lost. The responsibility for air pollution and thus the smog was divided between three Ministries: Health and Local Government; Housing and Environmental Regulation (later the Ministry of Housing and Local Government); and Fuel and Power. The last of these was also responsible for research in this area.

Pressure from the media, the National Smoke Abatement Society, public health doctors and questions in Parliament culminated in the appointment of a committee of enquiry in May 1953, with Sir Hugh Beaver as Chairman. With extraordinary haste, the committee reported in November 1953 (HMSO, 1953). It recommended that a public alert system should be introduced and that the wearing of smog masks (akin to surgical masks) should be encouraged to reduce the amount of particulate matter entering the respiratory tract. The most important recommendations were for the reduction of smoke from domestic chimneys, which were seen as the major cause of pollution because they were near the ground and concentrated in cities. Industrial emissions tended to be from tall chimneys of which there were comparatively few.

The Ministry of Housing and Local Government showed little interest in the problem, being preoccupied with floods on the East Coast and national programmes for housing construction. On the other hand the Ministry of Health reacted to the pressure for reforms and set up its own committee early in 1953 to investigate the medical aspects of the problem. The committee concluded in its report (Ministry of Health, 1954) that the irritants responsible for death and the increased incidence of respiratory illness in those suffering from respiratory or cardiac disorders were probably derived from the products of burning coal. The Ministry of Housing and Local Government showed no more interest in the deliberations of this committee than in those of the Beaver Committee.

The reports were well received but it seemed unlikely that the Government would act on their recommendations. There were already moves afoot to reduce the use of coal to limit the stranglehold that the miners had on the economy—central heating was becoming fashionable and nuclear power looked like becoming a reality—but the Government's hand was forced because, in response to the Beaver Committee report, Gerald Nabarro presented a Private Member's Bill to Parliament in December 1954. The support generated by this Bill led to the Clean Air Act of 1956 (for a more detailed account of the History of the Clean Air Act see Hall et al, 1975).

From the 1950s onwards, interest in the effects of air pollution grew. Studies of mortality and morbidity were undertaken to find out under what conditions and to whom air pollution caused harm and to determine which constituents of the pollution were the culprits. Hundreds of studies were mounted. Their quality was variable and their conclusions, as with those from most epidemiological studies which depend on value judgements of the evidence in hand, could be destroyed by intellectual purists. Epidemiological studies can demonstrate the qualitative effects of harmful agents but it is difficult to use them to arrive at precise dose-response relationships. The setting of standards therefore has to be accomplished by negotiation between the interested bodies. Nevertheless, it has been on epidemiological evidence that 'legislation for clean air has been based.

DEVOLUTION OF RESPONSIBILITY

The decision to legislate over air pollution from domestic chimneys differs from that of seatbelts in the implementation of the legislation was delegated to local authorities, and more importantly, the decision on whether to implement or not was left to local areas. Local agreement on the introduction of some policies is seen as important and the legislation was confined to enabling local authorities to act rather than dictating action to them. Fluoridation of water supplies has been left to the discretion of regional water boards and health authorities. In many cases, even where action is required, local authorities are left to determine local needs and the best means of meeting them. Such devolution is considered vital to the successful running of the health services. The NHS is organised to be administratively independent of central government. As a consequence, although the DHSS allocates funds to the 14 Regional Health Authorities (RHAs) which determine capital and general expenditure policies for the Districts within them, the District Health Authorities (DHAs) determine their own priorities for meeting local needs.

The policy of devolution leads to a number of conflicts of loyalties within the NHS. The key employees, and therefore the main users of NHS resources are the health professionals who work within it, the most prominent of whom are clinicians. In order to be free to act in the best interests of their patients, they are held accountable only to their patients for the care that is given. Clinical autonomy results in clinicians being their own managers acting within the broad policy guidelines laid down by the DHSS and within accepted medical practice. However, the NHS financed through general taxation is, as a whole, accountable to the Secretary of State responsible for health services. He in turn is ultimately accountable to the taxpayers as voters and to their representatives in Government who hold the public purse. Moreover, as indicated above each DHA is accountable to the local constituency it serves. This is demonstrated by the presence of elected members of the local authority on the DHA, along with appointees by the RHA and representatives of health professions and local university institutions.

Thus there is a three way division of accountability which can cause conflicts of interests. The NHS is accountable to the taxpayers through the members of Government for provision of the best possible care for the nation as a whole. The clinician is expected to achieve the best possible care for each patient and the NHS management is responsible for the best deployment of limited resources between all patients.

The broad objectives of the NHS as laid out in the legislation are too vague to form a basis for policy decisions: for example, they do not give any criteria by which health services should be allocated to individuals. The limited availability of resources means that some people will not be able to receive the care they need. For other policies, society, through its policy makers, determines which groups should receive particular resources, by defining eligibility criteria for receipt of services. Health care is allocated on the basis of need and in consequence clinicians are left to determine to whom resources should be allocated.

Where patients feel they have not received the best care because of maladministration they have the right to complain, although malpractice suits lie outside the NHS organisation. Community Health Councils (CHC) act as watchdogs to promote patient and public interests at District level, and behave similarly to other groups which protect consumer interests in nationalised industries. CHCs have the right to monitor their local health services and to complain about issues which relate to the non-clinical aspects of service provision. Individuals who wish to complain can use the CHC as a vehicle for action. Another pathway is also open to dissatisfied patients; the Health Service Commissioners or Ombudsmen can undertake investigations and make recommendations on patient complaints about administrative matters.

The conflict of preserving clinical freedom whilst maintaining the health service management interest in resource conservation is a perennial problem. Each doctor, in using health service resources for a patient, consumes resources which are then not available either for his other patients, or for other doctors' patients. Also the best use of resources for one patient is not necessarily the optimum use of resources for the community of patients or potential patients as a whole. To overcome this, the NHS has evolved a system of management which involves doctors and other professionals. There are a number of ways in which this is achieved. Representatives of health professions are included in both the team of officers responsible for running district health services and in the district policy making body, the DHA. In addition, committees made up of groups of professionals advise the officers and the policy makers. This involvement achieves three objectives: firstly, clinicians bring accurate and current knowledge of the clinical situation to bear on management decisions; secondly, clinicians are committed to the proposals for change through their participation in making decisions; and thirdly, the clinicians obtain an understanding of the impact of their work on the rest of the running of the health service.

Although the need for local flexibility reflected through a policy of devolution is obviously considered vital to the NHS, there is also concern about the maintenance of standards and comparability of intra-district care. Where a health district or local authority elects to consider a programme, it must be achieved within certain objectives which satisfy not only local but also national observers. In some cases guidelines are suggested, in others more rigid standards are applied as, for example, the levels of pollutants allowed in the atmosphere. These can be achieved either through definitive legislation or through Acts of Parliament which can confer decision making powers on Ministers, allowing them to issue statutory instruments or orders in council which can bind the health service to fulfil certain requirements.

CONCLUSION

No specific objectives exist to determine a universal model upon which policies for the prevention, diagnosis and treatment of illness can be built. On each occasion politically expedient actions have to be determined, the main aim of which is to achieve the most acceptable compromise for all interested parties. The parties involved differ according to the subject on which the decision is to be made, and can include professional bodies, industry and pressure groups championing specific causes.

In accordance with long historical tradition the Government remains wary of infringing the liberty of the individual, commerce or local government. The evidence to justify an intervention must be strong and political support great before a policy becomes acceptable. In general the Government has shown a reluctance to intervene in the lives of individuals, preferring to persuade them through education of the need to reduce risks to their health. Only recently, as evidence demonstrating the inability of some groups to change their behaviours emerges, are universal and sanctioning policies considered as possible actions. Where conflicting interests exist, such as those of the tobacco companies in the debate over reducing the amount of smoking, the economic and political feasibility of any action has to be carefully considered.

Where possible, decisions which do not require universal application are passed to local bodies to acquire local agreement. For example, it would not be acceptable in Britain at the current time for local authorities to decide whether their police forces should enforce the wearing of seatbelts. Administratively and organisationally this would not be feasible. However, the fluoridation of water supplies is appropriate for local decision making, for a number of reasons. Firstly the levels of fluoride contained in local water supplies vary from place to place and it would be difficult to prescribe precise amounts of fluoride to be added. Secondly, it is in general much easier for legislators to remove chemical agents than to prescribe their consumption. If in the future fluoride is found to have harmful effects, then the government of the day cannot be held wholly responsible for the damage that has occurred. All decisions made through powers conferred on local bodies by specific legislation are open to contest in the courts. Where legislation enables policy decisions to be taken, the policy must be subordinate to the legislative process which can alter or reverse the decisions taken.

Within the NHS, which is mainly concerned with the provision of health services, policies are created at national level and in most cases, implemented at the local level in accordance with locally determined needs and priorities. Respect for clinical freedom and protection of the doctor-patient relationship are considered to be of paramount importance so national policies to amend medical practice tend to be cautious and addressed to clinicians individually. This occurs either through the professional advisory machinery which links into the management system, or by informing the individual practitioners of recent research developments and the advice of the government's expert advisers. Local policies, especially those relating to changes in the uses of limited resources, can be generated by or negotiated with clinicians through the management system.

These policy decisions are not static. With increasing research, the state of knowledge changes, and with this attitudes and the resulting policies change. Economic features of decision-making also become increasingly important as more demands are created by improved technology for limited resources. Centralisation and increased central controls leading to greater uniformity for health related policies are not acceptable at the moment but there is no reason to prevent them from being introduced in the future. Policy is created by informed political beliefs. Epidemiological, social, medical and economic research contribute to changing ideas about what makes 'good' and 'acceptable' policy.

REFERENCES

DHSS 1974 Diet and coronary heart disease. Report of the Advisory Panel of the Committee on Medical Aspects of Food Policy (Nutrition) on Diet Relation to Cardiovascular and Cerebrovascular Disease. London

Goffman E 1963 Stigma: the management of spoiled identity. Prentice-Hall, Englewood Cliffs

Hall P, Land H, Parker R, Webb A 1975 Change, choice and conflict in social policy. Heinemann Educational, London

HMSO 1953 Interim Report of the Committee on Air Pollution. Cmnd 9011 (The Beaver Report) London

HMSO 1962 A hospital plan for England and Wales. Cmnd 1904 London

HMSO 1963 Health and welfare: the development of community care. Cmnd 1973. London

HMSO 1977a Prevention and health. Cmnd 7074. London

HMSO 1977b First report from the Expenditure Committee, session 1976/77. Preventive medicine, Volume I Report. London

HMSO 1979 Report of the Royal Commission on the National Health Service. Cmnd 7615. London

Jones K, Brown J, Bradshaw J 1978 Issues in social policy. Routledge and Kegan Paul, London

Journal of the Royal College of Physicians 1976 Vol 10, no 3 Prevention of coronary heart disease. Report of a Joint Working Party of the Royal College of Physicans of London and the British Cardiac Society

McNichol J 1980 The movement for family allowances 1918–45. Heineman Educational, London

Ministry of Health 1954 Mortality and morbidity during the London fog of December 1952. Report on Public Health and Medical Subjects. No 95. Report by a Committee of Departmental Officers and Expert Advisors Appointed by the Minister of Health. London

South East London Screening Study Group 1977 A controlled trial of multiphasic screening in middle age: results of the South East London screening study. International Journal of Epidemiology 6 (4): 357–63

Index